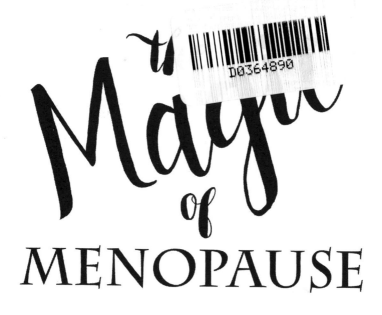

The Magic of

MENOPAUSE

A Holistic Guide to Get Your **Happy Back!**

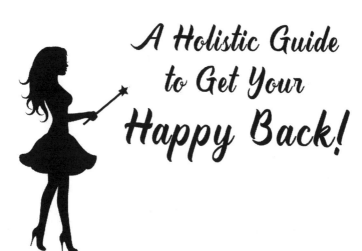

LORRAINE MIANO

The Magic of Menopause
A Women's Holistic Guide on How to Get Your *Happy* Back!

Copyright 2016 by LORRAINE MIANO

To contact the author or publisher, visit
INFINITEYOUHEALTH.COM

ISBN-10:1-944134-06-9
ISBN-13:978-1-944134-06-8
Printed in the United States of America

A Big Magical Thank You!

To my menopause sisters, for sharing their *Menopause Moments:* Jackie Fisher, Millie Bozek, Joanne DeLangie, Nan Maples, Linda Pukalo and Lori Anderson.

To my dear friend, Carla Payne, for sharing her extensive knowledge on Aging Life Care.

To my editor, Amanda Filippelli, and designer, Amie Olson, of Promoting Natural Health, for all of their hard work, guidance, suggestions, creativity, and especially for keeping me on track. You two rock!

To all of my family members, who always show their support for all I do: My three children, Nick, Jackie, and Rissy, their spouses Jayne, Kirk, and Dan; my parents, Al and Ro; my sisters, Denise and Marie, and their families. I love you all to the moon and back!

To my four grandchildren, Noah, Arabelle, Adelaide, and newborn Maxwell, for bringing so much joy to my heart and providing me with a reason to strive to live a sustainably healthy and long life!

And finally, to my dear hubby, Richard, who continues to show his love, support and pride in me, and who is willingly my "health" Guinea pig. You are my life. XXXOOO infinity more.

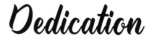

Dedication

*This book is dedicated
to the women in my life who,
through example, led me on my quest
for a life filled with purpose,
health & happiness,
especially my two grandmothers,
Marion and Caterina.*

Contents

Introduction

"You're going to be a Grandma."

WHAT?

When thrust upon you, these words bring a multitude of emotions ranging from pure joy and happiness ("I am going to be a grandmother!!!") to disbelief and dismay ("I am too young to be a grandmother!"). As if being in the midst of menopause wasn't enough to get the crow lines quivering, I was now being informed that I was acquiring a new title: GRANDMOTHER. At the time, the picture I envisioned in my head was one of an elderly lady in a house dress wearing an apron with her gray hair in a loose bun. Although it was a warm and endearing vision, it was most definitely NOT me! Add to this the fact that a hysterectomy was also scheduled in my very near future. I felt as though I had been pushed off the edge of the cliff into full tilt YOU-ARE-GETTING-OLD mode!

I was only forty-eight and a triple threat was thrust onto my doorstep. I immediately set out on my quest to find the fountain of youth, but not for the reasons you may think. Yes, of course I wanted glowing skin, a trim waistline, and as few laugh lines as possible, which is hard to do when you live amongst family comedians, although, side note: the laughing does help to build strong abs. However, what I wanted more than this was a future; a long and healthy future filled with Nonni, my "grandma" name, fitfully playing with the grandkiddies—tumbling, running, lifting, throwing, and all with the youthful glow of a body well-kept from the inside out!

Serendipity occurs frequently in my life, or maybe it is synchronicity. Either way, about eight years ago, just when menopause was hitting me full in the face, I was directed to a book that literally changed my life. The book is called *The Truth About Beauty* by Kat James. At that time, I was suffering from the usual annoying and disruptive menopausal symptoms of hot flashes, night sweats, mood swings, fatigue, vaginal dryness and weight gain. I was definitely lacking in the "happy" department. Although the book was not directly related to menopause, it led me on a journey of holistic health. It was there amongst Kat's glorious pages where I discovered that the simple act of changing my eating habits could literally change every aspect of my life. There was no reason to starve myself, go on a multitude of fad diets, or even partake in extreme exercising.

I started treating my body well with healthy nourishment and a regular simple exercise routine. It is as simple as eating what is good, not eating what is not, and making a few changes to some daily habits. What I found hit a chord with me. It was about getting *healthy*, not *losing weight*. Balanced hormones, a reduction of menopausal symptoms, weight loss, fewer wrinkles, glowing skin, fewer aches and pains, and more energy just happen to be the magical side effects. No quick fixes, but true lifestyle changes. I became passionate about sharing what I had learned, and eventually, at a point in my life where many would consider retiring, I found my calling—a career as an Integrative Nutrition Health Coach. Not only do I get to experience this great life filled with wonderful whole foods, exercise that I enjoy, and feeling absolutely fabulous, but I get to help others do the same!

I soon realized that, as a menopausal woman living in the twenty-first century, I still had thirty percent of my life ahead of me. That is a damn long time! That is an extremely long time to have to deal with the effects that menopause may wreak in our bodies and in our lives. I want to live my life to the absolute fullest! I don't want to have to deal with any symptoms that may keep me from doing just that. I want to help other menopausal women who are experiencing the effects of hormonal imbalances to have more energy, less stress, and to feel comfortable in their own skin. Ultimately, I would love for *you* to be able to live your life without limits! I want to help *you* live life the way you were meant to—with passion, purpose, and a healthy body and mind! Together we can help you find the happiness you may be missing! We will find the happiness you deserve!

You don't have to have grandchildren or have experienced a hysterectomy to feel or imagine the effects of menopause. We are reminded everyday about the "suffering" of the pause! Not half an hour goes by during prime time that there isn't a commercial by those big pharma pushers reminding you that you may need a pill to help with any number of the multitude of menopausal "symptoms" your body is plaguing you with. Anxiety, depression, hot flashes, thinning hair, mood swings, vaginal dryness, low libido, dry skin, wrinkles, weight gain, craving extremely salty potato chips, oh wait... Heck, if you weren't feeling low before the prime time perps assaulted your chill time, they've got their game down pat. "Ask your doctor about this med or that one, but please be aware, side effects include insomnia, nausea, diarrhea, fatigue, sleepiness, tremors, indigestion, suicidal thoughts, decreased libido, excessive sweating, anorexia, agitation, ejaculation failure (in case you had thoughts of sharing the drug with your spouse or partner)." WHAT?! The side effects are worse than the symptoms. You may need a new pill to cure you from taking the first pill. No, thank you!!!

I am here to tell you that the suffering need not happen! There are changes you can make right now in your life to keep those symptoms from rearing their ugly heads. This, more than any other time in your life, is yours to embrace and celebrate! There is magic in menopause! When you hear those words, "You're going through the changes," you can say, "Damn right I'm changing! I am becoming the woman I've always wanted to be!" Now is the time for the suffering to end!

Read on to see how you can get your *happy* back and live the magical life you crave!

My Two Grandmothers

Happy. Healthy. Dead. I remember when I first heard that phrase while training to become a health coach, I thought, "Wow, how morbid." But then I really stopped to think about the words. *Happy.* Yes, I want to be happy. I'd like to be constantly happy. Every day, always. *Healthy.* Yup, I'm all for that one too. *Dead.* Well, no, I'm not ready for that one yet. Not for a very long while. Why would "dead" be part of a health coach's mantra? Dead? I thought we were about helping people get healthy and live longer?! Then, it hit me. There is nothing else in between healthy and dead—no long drawn out diseases, no aching, fatigued, stressed body. Straight from healthy to dead. Yes! That is what I want.

I don't want to be on all sorts of meds. I don't want to be suffering from any ailments. I want to be active, fit, healthy, and enjoying every minute of every day. I, as most folks I know, would love to pass peacefully in my sleep at a ripe old age. Ideally, it would be after I met my purpose, fulfilled my dreams, saw my great- grandchildren married off. Living a sustainably healthy lifestyle could provide that possibility. Of course, when you mention this to some people, they retort, "Well, I am just going to enjoy my life! I'm going to eat and drink what I want! Do what I want! You could get hit by a bus tomorrow and it would all be for nothing." Well, yes, there is always the possibility of an accidental death. But how I see it, I would like to increase my odds of living a long, enjoyable life. And quite possibly, if you *are* fit and healthy, you could outrun that bus collision. Happy. Healthy. Dead. I'll take it.

As a mature woman who was on the brink of becoming a grandmother and experiencing some rather unpleasant menopausal symptoms, I often thought about my upbringing and the time I spent with my own grandparents. Growing up, I was fortunate to have two grandmothers and one grandfather. When comparing myself to my two grandmothers, I'd think about the state of their health, their lifestyles and habits.

Each of my grandmothers had such an impact on my life. Most of my fondest memories include them. I decided when I started having children that I was determined to be that type of grandparent when the time came. I wanted to be someone's fondest memory. I wanted to create moments to cherish—the kind of moments that can shape a life. Giving of yourself, the most positive parts of yourself to a loved one, is probably the most treasured gift you can bestow on them. Your time, your laughter, your positive ideals, and even your sweet, warm hugs are the things that children or grandchildren remember and treasure. I had these types of grandparents.

My two sisters and I always felt as though we were the most important people in the world to them. I can still hear the songs my Irish-German grandmother sang to us. To us, she was "Nanny." Her laugh was contagious. She and my grandpa would care for us during our school breaks at their apartment in the Bronx. We lived out on Long Island, or

The Island, as we called it. We loved those stays with Nanny and Grandpa. I could not tell you one material gift they ever gave us (excluding the boxes of candy that Grandpa would pick up at Grand Central Station on his trip home from the office). However, the time they shared with us, singing and playing games, or the fabulous places they would take us, like the Bronx Zoo, the circus, or Radio City for the Christmas show, are deeply embedded in the treasure box of memories in my heart.

Nanny also happened to be a smoker and a drinker—not an uncommon thing during the fifties and sixties. Although I don't ever recall her being overweight, I am now quite certain she probably suffered from MONW, or metabolically obese normal weight. This is where you are under lean but over fat, having not enough muscle and too much fat. She gave up smoking in her late sixties, but unfortunately, emphysema found its way into her life. Rather, it found its way into *our lives*. Nanny, who I loved and adored, was soon bed ridden, on an oxygen tank, and would live out the remainder of her life in a small 9x10 bedroom.

Emotions flood me as I write this. Both anger and sadness fill my heart when I grieve the loss of my Nanny. I grieve for those years I was unable to share my life with her. I am saddened when I think of the visits I made to see her. I would sit by her side for hours and talk, while she was unable to breathe without an oxygen tank. Rarely did she leave her bed. My grandfather would care for her, cook for her, and watch her wither away. I am angry that some simple lifestyle changes may have saved her life. She could have lived for many more years. My children might have heard her songs and her contagious laughter or felt her warm embraces and her unconditional love. Bed ridden, she could not come and be with me on my wedding day. My grandfather came, and my heart ached for him. He was unable to dance with the love of his life as we celebrated. She was not in my wedding pictures. I can only imagine the feelings she had that day as she lay in her bed, unable to watch the granddaughter she sang to, who she cradled and loved, walk down the aisle and into the arms of the love of her life. She passed away soon after my marriage, never to know my three beautiful children.

There was also my paternal Sicilian grandmother who we referred to as Grandma. She was widowed at the very young age of thirty-five, left with four boys, aged twelve and under, to raise during the Depression. They lived in the Bronx. She barely spoke English yet worked very hard to keep those boys on the straight and narrow. With the help of her widowed mother, they labored day and night by taking in sewing and bead embroidery. Those four boys each went on to serve their country, get married, and raise wonderful families. My grandma never dated or remarried.

My grandma was an emotionally strong woman who endured much in her life, from leaving her home of Palermo, Sicily at the age of sixteen to raising her four boys with little to no money. My dad was the youngest, and when he felt his mother shouldn't be living on her own anymore, he purchased a home with a small cottage on the property for her to live in. Prior to that time, Grandma would come and care for us in the summers so that Mom and Dad could work. I shared my bedroom with her. She slept on the trundle that pulled out from beneath my bed. It was the kind that lifted up to the height of the bed. We had so much fun on those summer nights. Grandma's broken English was the basis of some frequent amusement for us. All in good fun, we would give her some funny words to repeat, like "hippopotamus" or "Englebert Humperdinck." She laughed harder than we did no matter how many times we had her repeat the words.

It was during those night time laughing fests that Grandma introduced me to her rituals, or as I realize now, her self-care routines. She would begin by laying in the dark, telling me some stories from back home in Sicily, so descriptive that I could smell the lemons and hear the sounds of the city streets. As she told her stories, she would do her "exercises." First, she would take each wrist and turn them in circles several times to the left, then several more times to the right, one hand and then the other. Then circling arms would commence, followed by ankles, and lastly, her legs. When this routine was complete, the moisturizing ritual began. I believe it fluctuated between Noxzema and Vaseline. Grandma would massage the product onto her face and décolletage, followed by her arms and hands. This ritual was a nightly occurrence, no exceptions.

During that time, I was between ten and twelve years old. I can still smell the Noxzema when I recall the stories she shared with me. When you think of a Sicilian, you imagine a dark, olive-skinned person, someone who tans easily. However, my grandmother was raised to "never go in the sun!" She endured sunburn but one time in her life, and she was punished by her mother for allowing it to happen. As a lady, you were to keep your skin pure. Well, if ever there was a model for the ideal porcelain skin, it was my grandmother. She barely had any wrinkles and the texture and tone of her skin was magnificent! As teenagers in the seventies, my sisters and I often baked in the sun, and quite frequently, we doused ourselves in baby oil. We never needed the iodine addition that so many of our friends used. Sicilian genes were enough to give us that golden glow. Of course, that glow often did not come until after an extreme sunburn, which on occasion, was also blistering and peeling. What in the world were we thinking? We were literally frying our young skin! I could hear my grandma moaning as she watched us laying on our towels around the pool.

"Girls! What are you doing? You are going to ruin your skin!" she would lament in broken English.

We would just laugh and say, "Don't worry, Grandma. We will be okay!"

"No! No! It's not good!"

Of course, she was right, and my splotchy skin did pay the price. I have to say, my grandmother was ahead of her time. Or maybe we need to get *back* to the times she was from—simple and healthy skin care, pesticide-free and organically grown food, environmentally sustainable practices like deposit bottles and cloth shopping bags. I often refer to those times as "the good old days" much to my daughters' chagrin. Yet times did seem so much simpler and less "processed" then.

Grandma did suffer a bit with type 2 diabetes in her later years. I believe her sweet tooth for Stella D'oro cookies and love of pasta contributed to that. Her main nutrition, however, was a true Mediterranean diet complete with extra virgin olive oil, lots of fresh fruits, veggies, and lean meats. We were fortunate as children to be introduced to many foods that our friends never heard of or dreamt of trying—fava beans, escarole, calamari, and scungilli. She prepared some very interesting and tasty dishes! We still make many of them today and always think of her. Grandma lived to be almost ninety. She died peacefully in her sleep.

Now you've got a small picture of my grandmothers. As most grandchildren do, I came to be with them when they were in the prime of their menopause years. As a child of the baby boom generation, I don't ever recall my grandmothers talking about it or even visibly noticing any of the symptoms associated with what we are now told is "menopause."

I don't recall them fanning themselves or complaining about how warm they were. Quite possibly, this was due to their diets growing up during the earlier part of the twentieth century. Processed foods were not a part of their lives. The foods they ate were organic. Pesticides for crops and antibiotics for livestock did not come until the fifties and sixties, and the baby boomers are reeling from the effects of those toxins now.

Research suggests that women who are extensively exposed to common chemicals found in plastics, personal care items, household items, and the environment are likely to experience early onset menopause, as compared to women with lower exposures. Scientists suspect that these environmental chemicals are causing hormone disruption as well as gynecological diseases. Did you know that menopausal symptoms vary around the world and in different cultures? For instance, women in India report no significant menopausal symptoms other than menstrual changes. In Japan, the symptom most reported is shoulder stiffness, with hot flashes being very rare. Researchers suggest that there may be a direct link between diet and lifestyle habits, and their effect on hormones. One interesting suggestion is that western culture, which looks at menopause as an "ending," may determine a woman's experience with menopause, versus other cultures where menopause is looked upon as a time of new respect and freedom. All of this interesting information leads me to wonder: Could the changing landscape of our western environment be affecting our female health from puberty through menopause?

Spending a good portion of my childhood and young adult years with my grandmothers allowed me to observe the effect that their lifestyle choices played on their health and wellbeing during their menopausal years. My two grandmothers were two different people with different lifestyle habits. I wish that Nanny had taken better care of herself. Smoking cigarettes for a good portion of her life and excessive alcohol consumption took its toll on her. Watching her live out the last few years of her life bedridden, unable to breathe on her own, losing so many years that she might have spent with her loved ones truly broke my heart. I would have loved to have more time with her.

Grandma was my first inspiration for the benefits of simple exercise routines and skin care. Perhaps the fact that she took the time to care for herself with daily exercise and skin care rituals, as well as eating a healthy diet throughout her menopausal years, allowed her to live a healthy and enjoyable life well into her late eighties. Science proves that eating a well-balanced and healthy diet as well as following certain lifestyle habits will help you balance your hormones. This, in effect, will also keep your bones strong, enabling you to be physically active into your later years. Grandma somehow knew what she needed to do to stick around for a while. She successfully did so and was around for the births of close to ten great grandchildren.

I loved both of my grandmothers immensely and miss them dearly. They have provided the influence that drives my desire to live gustily, passionately, and with purpose. Together, for better or for worse, they are my inspirations for living a sustainably happy, healthy life; a life that I plan on sharing with my grandchildren and great-grandchildren for decades to come. I have seen first-hand the kind of life that can be experienced by taking simple steps to care for myself. I am determined to make my years of "the change" the very best years of my life, bringing all of you lovely ladies along with me for the ride!

As Lauren Bacall once said during her midlife, "I'm not a *has-been*, I'm a *will-be.*"

ONE

Let the Party Begin

Welcome to your magical menopausal life! Yes, you heard that correctly. This is your magical, wonderful, fantastic and fabulous life, and I can prove it to you.

There is a reason you picked up this book. Maybe you are in the midst of menopause and you are feeling overwhelmed with annoyingly persistent symptoms like hot flashes, mood swings, weight gain, anxiety—all of those things that are often made light of in jokes or mixed company. Possibly, you are feeling depressed and/or anxious. Quite possibly, you are peri-menopausal and you don't understand what is happening to your body. You may be experiencing the social stigma that comes with the perception of menopause. Misconceptions, ageism and sexist views may find you withholding from sharing your emotions and concerns. Your support system may be lacking. You are wondering if this is normal. Is this what life is going to be like from now on? Is there a chance I can change what is happening to me? Am I alone in this? Can I get some relief? Can I get my HAPPY back????

I will show you how you can truly embrace this time of change, accept it, and actually enjoy and celebrate this natural and magical process of your life.

So, you may ask, what is so magical about menopause?

Women are conditioned to believe that menopause is a stage of life that is to be feared and even avoided if possible. They are often left confused and apprehensive when presented with misinformation or certain "myths" about "the change." Some of these myths include assuming that weight gain is inevitable or that your sex drive will most definitely decrease. This can lead to confusion and even anxiety. Recently, I read an article that even suggested that women over the age of fifty feel as though they become "invisible." They are made to feel as though they are not vital any longer. They are no longer fertile and may feel less attractive. These feelings may come in stages, as in the first time you aren't asked to show your ID when purchasing a bottle of wine or when you are offered the senior discount at the movie theater. This "feeling" may even extend to the workplace.

Although great strides are being made to understand and support pregnant women, menopausal women may be left in the dust. The average age that menopause occurs is fifty-one, with symptoms lasting between two to ten years. This is an age where many women are still active in the workforce. About twenty percent of the American workforce (about twenty-seven million women) experience menopause. For many women, stress levels increase during menopause and there are times when menopausal symptoms can interfere with work. Having heavy workloads and inflexible schedules can add even more stress. Frequent hot flashes or other physical symptoms can lead to embarrassment. Women may feel harassed, negativity, and even ridicule from others in the workplace. The fact that women experiencing menopause may not want to admit they are going through it, and men are uncomfortable talking about it, makes for an even more uncomfortable work place.

Fear, anxiety, confusion, and myths do not have to define your menopausal experience. Even if you are currently experiencing terrible symptoms or have a fear of the menopausal years, I am here to tell you that with some self-care and a little guidance, you can experience, what I call, the magic of menopause. You will feel better. You will look fantastic. You will love your life! You will get your *happy* back! After all, if you take care of yourself, follow some simple lifestyle habits, and have a positive outlook, you may never even find a lapse in your *happiness!* Even if you are currently in your premenopausal years and not experiencing any unpleasant symptoms yet, by following the holistic suggestions in this book now, I can guarantee that you may find your menopause years to be the happiest years you've ever had. Can't you just hear Pharrell Williams singing the soundtrack of your life?

Perimenopause is a natural progression of life. It is not a disease or something to be "cured." The most beneficial way to deal with the symptoms of menopause is to be ready for them. By this, I mean be of a healthy body in the physical as well as emotional and psychological sense. You can begin by embracing this time of your life. A positive attitude does wonders for creating a healthy body. Use the acronym H.O.P.E.: Have Only Positive Expectations. By *expecting* to be happy, more than likely, you will be on your way to actually *being* happy.

Be prepared to do some good work here. You have to invest the time in yourself. As your menopausal fairy godmother, I would love to just wave a wand, declare I am a miracle maker, and sprinkle magic dust all over you. Nothing would make me happier then to provide you with your *happy*. The truth is, though, this will take some time and effort on your part. But honey, you are worth it! Every squat, four mile walk, energizing green smoothie, and meditating moment will fill your *HAPPY* bucket. Enough of these moments will have your bucket overflowing will all kinds of *happy*!

Our life is what we make of it, so I want you to make a commitment to yourself: "I will have a magical life." Say it again and write it down. You can't help but smile when you say it. Better yet, say, "I will *LIVE* a magical life." There. You put it out in the universe. Now go and make it happen.

"But how?" you ask. "I'm not feeling magical at all. My hot flashes, plump belly, irritable moods, anxiety, hair loss, lack of energy, lack of sleep, lack of libido, and dry vagina all tell me... 'Magical?' I can think of a few choice words for what I am experiencing. This is as far from magical as you can get."

I am here to tell you that you have it in you! You will find that working from the inside out will give you a life you could only imagine. You can live the life you crave! Follow my simple guidelines, do some good work, and stardust will be swirling all around you. You *will* discover the magic of menopause.

Think of a woman or women in your life who you admire and hold in high esteem. It may be someone famous or even your next door neighbor. What is it about her that you admire? Her confidence? The way she carries herself? Her accomplishments? Her wit and humor? Her intelligence? Her skills?

What is the age of this woman? Is she in her twenties? Thirties? Probably not, right? More than likely she is a woman in her forties, fifties, or even sixties and beyond. She is a woman who has experienced life and has found her purpose. She is a woman who is comfortable in her own skin. You might look at her and think, "I'd like to be more like her, to have her confidence, her energy, to be happy with myself." I am here to share with you that you are not alone.

That fact that there is a stigma attached to menopause (in the sixties, Dr. Robert A. Wilson referred to menopausal women as "crippled castrates" in his book, *Feminine Forever*) often effects the way women look at themselves during "the change." Our thoughts and perceptions of menopause, along with the physical changes that are occurring, could ultimately determine the quality of the experiences we have during this time. If we look at menopause as a "natural plague" (also Dr. Wilson's words), then chances are our experience with it will be quite different then a woman who considers it a "new beginning" in her life. You may be anxious or fearful about the fact that you are aging. You may feel that there are limitations and restrictions to what you are able to do at this point. I want you to believe in yourself. You are a magnificent human being who is quite capable of anything that you put your mind to. You have strength, determination and character! You have a third of your life ahead of you. That is plenty of time to make your mark in this world. That is enough time to pursue your passions, follow your dreams, and make a difference wherever you put your two feet.

We are conditioned to think that youth is where it's at. Look younger! Feel younger! BE YOUNGER! I am here to tell you that it is not about being younger. It is about being happier. It is about being healthier—happier and healthier in mind, body, and spirit, having more confidence and being comfortable in your own skin. You can take better care of those around you by taking better care of yourself. This is not being selfish. There is a saying: "Give your loved ones the best of you, not what's left of you!" How absolutely true this statement is. As women, we are naturally nurturers. Often, we are concerned more for others' welfare before our own. This can take a lot of energy, physically as well as mentally, and ultimately, emotionally. We are often left drained. This is especially the case for women who are "in the middle," that sandwich generation who is caring for our aging parents as well as our adult children who are struggling to get on their feet.

This is a time in your life that you should embrace. This could be the time in your life that you've been waiting for, anticipating with glee! I can see your face right now. You have an incredulous smirk on your face, don't you? You are reading these words right now and thinking, "This woman is out of her mind." Well, what if I told you that these could be the absolute best years of your life? Yes, of your life! There are so many positives to being in the pause! You can wear white pants any day! All day! Whenever you want! (Even after Labor Day if your little ol' heart so desires!) That's right, NO MORE PERIODS!!! You get to save a few bucks on tampons and pads! Think about how liberating this is. You can leave your house anytime you like and not have to worry about that unexpected sudden wet gush as you sit down in the booth at your favorite restaurant, then having to run off to the ladies' room or even home! Oh, and what about SEX?! You can have sex anytime you want with no worries of pregnancy! Now, how liberating is that? You may even enjoy it more without the worry! What about those damn migraines? And PMS? Most women can say bye-bye to those hormonal throbbing headaches and mood swings after menopause! This is what famous American anthropologist Margaret Mead referred to as "postmenopausal zest." This is the time in your life when the monthly annoyances and inconveniences of having a period, PMS, cramping and birth control are in your rear view mirror. You may find a sudden burst of new energy and excitement in your life. You may find yourself re-evaluating different aspects of your life, especially at an emotional and psychological level. This is what the experience of a re-birth or a whole new beginning feels like. This is when you may decide to pursue a dream you've been keeping on the back burner, starting or changing your career, or even a relationship that is not serving you well. You may even decide that now is the time to become your healthiest and happiest self.

This just might be the time for you to shine! Find that purpose! Take a quantum leap! Menopausal women can feel more confident and empowered. Your families are grown and on their own. You have more time to pursue your goals and desires. You should have more time for self-love and care!

You can nurture those in your life, while also nurturing and caring for yourself. Remember, this is not being selfish. It is a matter of survival. Think of it as survival of the fittest. The fittest as being healthy, happy, active, and full of purpose.

If you are at a point in your life where you are fortunate to have found your purpose or to have fulfilled your dreams, now is the time to expand and live life to its fullest potential.

If you are still searching for your purpose, your menopause years are the absolute perfect time to discover or re-discover yourself. You have more freedoms, possibly more financial security. You may find yourself with more free time to pursue goals. You should feel more comfortable in your own skin. Some women I've coached have found themselves recently single (some by choice, others not). Quite understandably, this could be a challenging situation, emotionally as well as financially. You are a strong being. You can survive. You can succeed. You can be *happy*.

There is a quote by Earl Nightingale that I love: "Never give up on a dream just because of the time it will take to accomplish it. The time will pass anyway."

As a woman who is in the midst of her menopausal years, you may find yourself succumbing to the stereotypes and misconceptions that society has ignorantly placed upon us. It does not mean that you are old or nearing the end of your life. For goodness sake, you have at least a third of your life ahead of you! Just think of the contributions you still have to make, the passions you can still pursue, the dreams that have yet to be fulfilled. You may find these to be the most productive years of your entire life! Here are just a few steps to follow to get you on your way to living the life that will have you exploding with happiness:

Education: Learning should be a lifetime goal. Do what you love, love what you do. If you are stuck in a career that is not serving you well or you just want to make a change, now is the time. Possibly you were a stay-at-home mom like me, and feel that now is your time to shine. There are so many opportunities out there for you. With online education options, it is easier than ever to find your perfect career. If you aren't sure of what you want to do, take a vocational test to see where your strengths lay. Is there a hobby that you love? Turn it into a career! If you are creative, there are so many ways to promote and sell your art and crafts: Etsy, Pinterest, Bonanza, or create a Facebook page. If you already have an idea for your own business, but feel you lack business skills, take a course on how to run a business or how to be an entrepreneur. The world is at your fingertips. Google is your friend. If you don't have the funds to pay for an education, you can seek financial aid and scholarships. There are ways to eliminate those obstacles and let your dream shine!

1. **Volunteer.** If you are at a point in your life where you may be financially stable and are feeling fulfilled with your career, or you may even be ready to retire, you can find new purpose through serving others. According to the Corporation for National & Community Service, "There is a strong relationship between volunteering and health: those who volunteer have lower mortality rates, greater functional ability, and lower rates of depression later in life than those who do not volunteer." Where do your strengths lay? Are you a handy person? Maybe an organization like Habitat for Humanity could use your skills. Or perhaps you'd like to build homes for veterans. Do you love children? What about volunteering at a local hospital to cuddle babies? Often times, babies are too sick or small to go home right away. They may be in the neonatal unit for weeks. Families cannot sit by their bedside for weeks on end as they may have other children at home. Baby cuddlers fill this void. Cuddling babies calms them and aids in their early development. You can go to the other end of the spectrum and visit with seniors at assisted living or skilled care facilities. Spend some time playing games, reading, or just chatting with some elderly folks who could use your good company. Does your heart lay with the less fortunate? What about volunteering at the local food bank or shelter? Do you love animals? You could volunteer at an animal shelter or foster pets in your home. By volunteering, you are filling a void in someone else's life, and by doing so, you are filling one in your own as well. "Your talent is God's gift to you. What you do with it is your gift back to God." -Leo Buscaglia

2. **Creativity.** Have you dreamed of playing an instrument or maybe singing? Why not take some lessons now? Do you love painting or drawing, but never found the time for it? Now is the time! What about learning a new language? Do you love to write? Maybe you've got a book waiting to explode from your fingertips. In the words of George Eliot, "It is never too late to be what you might have been."

3. **Teach.** What do you know? What do you excel at? Share your gifts. You could teach a class or workshop at the local YMCA or community center. What about the local community college? Maybe tutoring?

   "A teacher affects eternity; he can never tell where his influence stops." -Henry Brook Adams

4. **Exercise/Health:** Do you have a specific exercise that you love or excel at? Yoga, Pilates, Zumba, or Tai Chi? Why not become certified and make it a career? What about a holistic practitioner? Acupuncturist, reiki practitioner, reflexologist, aromatherapist, health coach, masseuse? You reap the benefits of a healthy lifestyle while helping and encouraging others to do so too!

5. **Clubs/Groups:** Maybe you find yourself at a point in your life where you are ready to retire, but want to find things of interest to fill your time. Why not join a club of some sort? There are book clubs, running, walking, and swim clubs. Maybe Bible study groups or even a support group may be of help to you: grief share or women's health. Maybe you love music and either sing or play an instrument or both? Why not start

a musical group for fun? I have several friends in their fifties who have done this and find it is one of the greatest joys of their lives. Music is the universal language. The psychological and emotional benefits of belonging to a group are tremendous. *The 7 Amazing Benefits of Joining a Club,* according to All Women's Talk, are "making new friends, increasing your knowledge (learning a new subject), regular activity, fitness (if you join some sort of sports club or gym), discounts (The club often arranges discounts for its members. These can cover everything from cultural activities to special rates if you shop at local businesses. Discounts are also often available for items that you need for the club's activities.), events (leading to a packed social calendar), and networking (great, especially if you own a small business, to possibly meet a new partner, or make new friends)."

Part of finding purpose, activity, happiness, *a life*…is getting out of your chair, off the couch, and out of your house! The opportunities are endless. Menopause does not define us. We are strong, capable, and worthy. Discover your interest, your love, your gift, and you will be one step closer to getting your *happy* back!

"The Meaning of life is to find your gift.
The purpose of life is to give it away."

-Pablo Picasso

CREATING MAGICAL MOMENTS

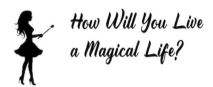

How Will You Live a Magical Life?

You are a fabulous woman who deserves to live a magical life! Having a daily reminder will help you on your way to actually living it! Cut out the following page and place it somewhere that you will be sure to see it every day—your bathroom mirror, beside your bed, your refrigerator, or your desk. Look at it daily. Read it out loud. You will be on your way to living the life you deserve! A happy, magical life!

I Will Live a Magical Life!

-Your Menopause Fairy Godmother
The Magic of Menopause

GRATITUDE JOURNAL

Take the time to use the next pages to discover your interest, your love, and your gift.

_____

_____

_____

_____

_____

_____

_____

_____

_____

_____

_____

_____

_____

_____

_____

_____

_____

_____

_____

_____

_____

_____

_____

_____

_____

_____

_____

_____

_____

_____

_____

_____

_____

_____

_____

_____

_____

_____

_____

_____

_____

_____

_____

_____

_____

_____

_____

TWO

Stress & Anxiety: Bye-Bye!

Unless you've experienced extreme anxiety, it's hard to understand exactly what it feels like. I am guilty of being one of those people who couldn't understand, be sympathetic, or who thought, "Just get over it." I want to sincerely apologize to anyone in my life who I may have been dismissive to when they were experiencing anxiety. At the age of fifty-six, I experienced my first anxiety attack. It wasn't until I had that feeling of, "What the hell is happening to me??" did it hit me full in the face. I was experiencing what I now refer to as "that evil monster." This was the kind of anxiety that leaves your heart pounding, your body shaking, and your mind racing with uncontrollable thoughts. I truly thought I was having a heart attack. I couldn't seem to catch my breath. The feeling in my gut reminded me of that feeling you get on the downward slope of a roller coaster, but it just wouldn't stop. I couldn't eat. I couldn't sleep. I could not control my thoughts.

On some level, many women, I believe, hold anxiety within the confines of their multitasking, nurturing (of everyone but themselves), and worrisome bodies. I am sure that I did for years. It rears its little ugly head in many different disguises, some of which include ADD, PMS, IBS, M&Ms…oh wait.

According to UCLA psychiatrist and anxiety expert, Dr. Jason Eric Schiffman, who is affiliated with the UCLA Anxiety Disorders Program and Anxiety.org, the connection between hormonal changes and anxiety and panic attacks is strong, especially during the peri-menopausal period, where women are more likely to experience the evil monster. Once menopause passes, many women find that their anxiety will decrease. There may also be other factors that can contribute to anxiety during menopause, such as an increase of physical symptoms or negative life events.

Sometimes we don't realize what is happening to us. Even more than this, we don't realize just what "anxiety" is physically doing to our female bodies. This is especially true as we approach middle-age and menopause. Changing hormones, physical and emotional changes, along with an increase in stress levels can lead to anxiety and depression in some women. The inability to "cope" with stress during the week before a menstrual cycle (PMS) can often lead to feeling more anxious. There have also been studies linking a decrease in estrogen levels during menopause with cognitive and memory dysfunction and having difficulty concentrating. These can mimic ADD symptoms, or in the case of women who may already have ADD/ADHD, can worsen their symptoms.

Most scientists agree that anxiety contributes to the onset of irritable bowel syndrome (IBS), also known as spastic colon. Some of the symptoms include diarrhea, constipation, bloating, gastrointestinal discomfort, and erratic bowel movements. Other factors may contribute to IBS, but anxiety is considered one of the main reasons.

There may also be the added worries of an aging body, caring for our parents, adult children, or both, and the frustration of possibly having friends and family members that can't understand what you are experiencing and going through.

My first anxiety attack occurred soon after the death of one of my closest and dearest friends, Candy. Candy and I met when my husband and I moved our family from Long Island, New York to Cary, North Carolina in the early nineties. We moved into a small colonial in a cul-de-sac in a growing community. Candy was the first neighbor to greet me. She was a cute, bubbly pixie with a southern twang, long blonde hair, a beautiful smile, and a great laugh. We instantly became friends. I was the dark haired, ethnic looking one (see Sicilian) with the Long Island accent counterpart to our dynamic duo.

As the moving van pulled into our new home, Candy was quick to invite us all over for lunch, knowing we'd be too busy to get it for ourselves. My three kids and husband, Rich, headed over while I checked in the furniture with the movers. She, of course, sent over a plate for me. This was at the end of summer, and soon the kids were off to school, and the two of us stay-at-home moms found time for what would become our weekly ritual—a stop at the drive-thru coffee shop, Jitters (a truly new concept, pre-Starbucks). Candy would get a vanilla latte and I'd have a café mocha (even our coffees resembled us!). Then, off we'd embark on a day of shopping, sometimes for clothes or items for the kids, other times to peruse the isles at the new Lowes food store.

We soon realized that we had grown up on opposite sides of the country—she in Texas, me in New York—basically living the same lives. We were the same age (Candy was older by a month). We loved Donny Osmond, The Jackson Five, and David Cassidy while growing up. We were those sweet and innocent twelve-year-old girls, enjoying a simple life in the early seventies.

Over the years, we travelled together to New York several times to visit my family—the two moms and a carload of five kids (her two, and my three), sixties music blasting in the car as we all sang and danced in our seats. We shared the same pullout sofa at my sister's home and laughed and giggled all night like two pre-teens at a sleep-over. Several times, we even brought our daughters to see The Monkees in concert. We all had a blast! It was wonderful to share a piece of our childhood with them.

Our connection was real. Candy and I had a bond that kept us connected over the course of 20+ years, even after we each moved from the cul-de-sac to different towns, thirty minutes apart. We vacationed together, we shopped together, and we laughed and cried together. As our children grew up, our weekly coffee and shopping expeditions turned into biannual ones and we would meet at the local mall. We found that we sat and chatted more (we had months of family info to catch up on) than we shopped. At the end of the day, we would hug and say goodbye at our usual spot in the parking lot behind Macy's and be on our way. Our "therapy" sessions were enough to tide us over until the next time.

This was girlfriend time—laugh until we cried or cry until there was nothing left to do but laugh time. Better than any therapy you could pay for. Every woman should have, at the very least, one of these types of girlfriends.

On December 13th, 2014, my most precious friend lost her self-less, courageous, ten-month battle with pancreatic cancer. She passed with her loving family by her side. Her husband would tell me later that not once did she ever worry about or feel sorry for herself. Her only concern was for her family, her husband of over thirty years, her son and her daughter. A true nurturer. Always. I am convinced...even still.

I wept. No! I sobbed for days. Gut wrenching, uncontrollable sobs. I couldn't speak of Candy without my voice wavering, a huge lump engulfing my throat. I already missed my friend, my partner in crime. Soon my thoughts were consumed with worry for her children. They were only in their twenties. They would not have their mom now as they found their way. Their grief became my own. There was so much about their loss that tore me up inside. Her daughter had lay in bed with her mom when her body was too weak to do anything else, and planned her wedding. An engagement had not even occurred yet. I learned from my daughter that Candy and her daughter planned her potential wedding, knowing (but hoping against all odds) that she most likely would not be there to share in her day.

These were the thoughts that gripped my heart, and ultimately, my physical being. I thought I was having a heart attack. I couldn't catch my breath. My fight-or-flight response continually rolled in my gut. I felt like I was falling. My mind was racing. My thoughts became morbid, depressed, and uncontrollable. What in the world was happening to me??

My sweet, concerned husband took me to an Urgent Care where I was hooked up to all kinds of equipment and an EKG was performed. Bloodwork was done. Questions were asked.

"Were you recently under a lot of stress?"

My simple answer was, "Uh, well, yes, I think. My best friend just passed away a couple of weeks ago."

On the inside, it was more like a screaming voice, "Yes!! My best friend, the friend who helped me raise my kids, shared all my secrets, laughed with me, cried with me, the friend who won't be there for her children's weddings or the birth of her grandbabies, my dearest, closest girlfriend will no longer be meeting me in the parking lot at Macys or giving me a big hug, a big smile, or tell me, 'Love to the family!'"

I am brought back to reality.

"Mrs. Miano, I believe you are experiencing severe anxiety."

I found it hard to believe. Me? Anxiety? I was of the belief that I had it all together. I was an emotionally strong person. Anxiety was not a part of my life. Yet I knew something was going on in my body. In my mind. In my life. Although I had previously experienced grief due to the death of my elderly grandparents and uncles, it was somehow expected and easier to accept. I had never felt the loss I found myself now experiencing—the loss of someone I shared so much of my life with, such a special friend who was such a big part of my child-rearing years. We had just stepped into the time in our lives where our children were all on their own and beginning their own adult lives. Each of us was experiencing the bittersweet effect that you feel as a woman who, after raising your children, now watched as they spread their wings to soar into the next part of their story. We, too, were on the verge of our next chapter. Although we, along with our spouses, were not quite at the point of retirement, we still shared our dreams of what that would look like for each of us in the future. Candy talked about retiring to the mountains, while I shared that it would depend on where all my kids ended up living. We would laugh about our "menopause brains" and the things that we would misplace or forget. Although we were both in the midst of "the change," and one of us would often break into a sweaty hot flash on one of our visits, we truly celebrated the fact that we were on the precipice of a new beginning; a new beginning with our husbands, our independence, and our new dreams. I loved being around Candy's energy. We always lifted each other up. I will forever miss our times together.

So, *this* is what anxiety feels like. One of my first thoughts was of guilt. How could I have been so dismissive of those who were fighting this evil monster? I suddenly felt compassion for those who had been suffering for years from panic and anxiety attacks. There are several who are very close to me.

It is such an uncontrollable feeling of unease and a kind of depression. What I did know was that I would do anything to rid myself of what I was experiencing and feeling. That is, anything constructive and productive. At that point in my life, I am certain that my hormones were out of balance. I am quite sure this contributed to what was happening to me. Combining a traumatic event with hormonal imbalance, along with all of the other normal stresses in my life, the evil anxiety monster said, "Boom! Here I am!"

During my first visit to the Urgent Care, the doctor sent me home with a four-day supply of Valium and insisted I make an appointment with my primary care physician. I followed his instructions. I had not slept for more than two to three hours per night for several days and was feeling desperate for relief. I did as I was directed and used two

Valiums per day for four days. Yes, it relieved my symptoms for a few hours. I was able to sleep.

I went to my primary care doctor who, after a long talk and examination, recommended I take an anti-anxiety med for at least a year so that there would be no chance of the anxiety returning. Evidently, she said, this could happen. I was NOT a happy camper. This was not what I wanted to hear. She also prescribed a generic form of Xanax for use in extreme situations for panic attacks. She warned me it is highly addictive and to use it infrequently.

I had already determined in my mind that I was not going to use it at all, smiled, and said, "Well, I am a holistic health coach, and really didn't want to take any meds." I always, even before anxiety, wanted to take the holistic and nutritional route when it came to taking medications, using them only as a last resort.

She highly suggested I consider the meds. I reluctantly agreed and left.

I knew that I did not want to experience the anxiety I had been going through and discussed my options with my husband. I considered the meds briefly, and in the end, together, we decided I would do some good work and figure out a more holistic course of action to "cure" my symptoms. At least I would try this first. I had heard so much about the negative side effects of some of these anti-anxiety meds, from physical to psychological, and was concerned, if not fearful to go this route.

The point of me telling you my story, of the gripping feelings that controlled my life for that brief time is because, as a menopausal woman, you may experience anxiety that effects your life. Often times it comes on during the menopausal years, and can be triggered by hormone imbalances, as well as certain events in our lives. As women, we may often suppress feelings of anxiety, leaving them to manifest into physical symptoms in our bodies. I want to share with you how I holistically relieved my symptoms of severe anxiety and continue to do so to this day. However, I will add a caveat here. Although I feel the methods I used worked for me, I understand the benefits of some meds when treating some folks dealing with psychological issues. I am not diagnosing or prescribing. I am, however, suggesting that holistic protocols may possibly work for you if you have anxiety. You should, however, always check with your doctor before taking any supplements, especially if you are currently taking any medications or other supplements.

So, this is how I got my happy back (as it pertains to anxiety):

I used Google to research holistic methods to cure my anxiety. I found a fabulous online course from the Calm Clinic (money well spent). The course is called "Recovery Formula for Women" and is set up in weekly modules. Each week, you are offered behavior modifications to follow to help you overcome your anxiety. Besides grief counseling, this course was probably the most significant thing I did to combat my anxiety. These two things actually help you get to the root of what is causing your anxiety, and fix it at its source.

Grief counseling, or counseling in general, in the event of tragic or disturbing events in your life is one of the best things you can do for yourself. It allowed me to speak from my heart about what I was going through without feeling any judgement. If you think you could use or need counseling, ask for recommendations from people you know, whether it be a friend or healthcare provider. If you see a counselor and feel that they just don't click with you, seek out a different one. You'll want to feel comfortable about sharing your concerns with someone you can trust. If money is an issue, there are many free counseling groups that you can find in your area. Most places of worship have some sort of program. You can search for a grief share group in your area as well.

Gratitude journaling was a life saver. Focusing on and appreciating all of the good in our lives provides us with the ability to open ourselves up to more abundance. If you begin each day with writing down the things that you are grateful for, it has set your tone for the day in the most positive way you could ever imagine. Often in the evenings, especially just before bedtime, while we are laying there, going over all of the things we must get accomplished and the worries we can't let go of, taking out a pen and paper and again writing down what we are thankful for provides us with a sense of peace and gratitude that can release us of the anxieties that hold our bodies and minds in their evil grip. Just start by writing down five things you are grateful for. Do it for thirty days and experience the difference it will make in your life.

To help with the relief of your symptoms, while learning how to cure your anxiety, you may want to use the following:

Supplements: I truly believe supplements were life savers for me. They are such a great support for women's health, especially as it pertains to stress and anxiety. Be sure to check with your healthcare provider before starting any supplements.

Vitamin B Complex: Consists of B1, B2, B3, B5, B6, B7, B9 and B12. These vitamins play an important role in our bodies. Vitamin B1, or thiamine, helps with strengthening the body when under stress as well as boosting the immune system. Vitamin B6 is responsible for helping the body make certain hormones and neurotransmitters (chemicals) in the brain, as well as helping to boost immune system functioning. B vitamins are responsible for metabolizing fat and protein, as well as helping the body convert food into glucose. This provides the body with energy. They are also responsible for helping with healthy nervous system functioning.

Fish Oil: Several studies have shown that the omega-3 in fish oil helps with mood disorders and depression. Interestingly, according to studies by Joseph Hibbeln, MD, a psychiatrist at the National Institute of Health, depression is on the rise in the United States, possibly due to our health conscious effort to reduce the amount of saturated fats and cholesterol in our diets. As Americans eat less of the good sources of omega-3, like red meat and eggs, they are increasing their intake of polyunsaturated fats, like soybean, corn and sunflower oils, which are lower in omega-3.

Check with your healthcare provider before taking a fish oil supplement, as omega-3 may worsen some conditions such as heart disease.

Magnesium: Low levels of magnesium in the body can lead to anxiety. There are so many benefits to taking a magnesium supplement. This supplement helps keep your blood pressure normal as well as keeps your bones strong. If you use PPI's (proton pump inhibitors) for treatment of acid reflux, such as Nexium, Prilosec or Prevacid, chances are your magnesium levels may be effected. I highly recommend using the very popular CALM by Natural Vitality, which is a powder that you mix with warm or hot water for a soothing drink. It is made from magnesium citrate and magnesium ascorbate and comes in several flavors like raspberry lemonade or orange. I like to take this just before heading to bed. This type of magnesium can act as a laxative so be sure to follow the directions and start with a small amount, building up to the recommended dosage. Another type of magnesium I like is the High Absorption 100% Chelated Magnesium by Doctor's Best. This does not have the laxative effect. It comes in pill form (albeit they are the size of horse pills!). This is elemental magnesium chelated with the amino acids glycine and lysine. Glycine has been shown to be an efficient carrier for minerals that facilitate absorption in the intestinal tract. Glycine is used by the body to form collagen, a key protein in cartilage and connective tissue. Lysine is an essential amino acid that assists gastric function. It is non-GMO, vegan, and gluten-free. Either type of magnesium supplement is beneficial. It's all a matter of what you prefer.

L-Theanine: This amino acid is found mostly in green and black tea. You can purchase it as a supplement, but should look for those made with Suntheanine. People diagnosed with anxiety have found that it helps by inducing a relaxing effect without causing drowsiness. It is also used to prevent Alzheimer's disease as well as to lower blood pressure, and has been granted GRAS (generally regarded as safe) status by the FDA.

Chamomile/Lavender Tea: I drink several cups of this tea daily for its soothing effect. There are many other types of herbal teas that can help soothe your anxiety as well, such as passionflower, kava, and peppermint.

Probiotics: Recent studies show a direct connection with your gut bacteria and your brain. Researchers have found evidence that a balance of your gut bacteria may do more for your mood than any other contributing factor. Taking a good probiotic as well as consuming probiotic foods will do wonders for your anxiety and depression. Some great probiotic foods are fermented veggies (such as sauerkraut, pickles and kimchi), Kefir (a kind of liquid yogurt drink), and kombucha tea.

To help further with your symptoms, reduce or remove the following list of items that can cause or exacerbate anxiety:

Caffeine: This stimulant can trigger your fight-or-flight response, which can make anxiety worse and trigger an anxiety attack.

Wine/alcohol: You may turn to a glass of wine or other alcoholic beverage to "soothe" your daily stress or nervousness, however, increased consumption of alcohol could actually increase your anxiety.

News programs: Of course you want to stay informed about what is occurring in our world, however, by limiting your exposure to the abundance of negative media we are bombarded with on a daily basis during times of extreme stress and anxiety in your own personal world, you can reduce the effects it will have on your personal health. I am not suggesting you discontinue listening to the news, just reducing it to a comfortable, bearable level.

Violent media: In much the same way that negative news stories can impact your mood, you may want to limit the number of violent movies and shows you view to keep your anxiety and stress levels to a minimum.

Too much computer and/or device time: This is linked to an increase in anxiety and depression, especially if you are using more than one device at a time.

You may want to add the following to improve your mood and reduce anxiety:

Exercise: You need to get out and move! Exercise helps to reduce anxiety and improves your mood! Just twenty minutes of exercise when you are feeling anxious can do wonders!

Breathing and Meditation: These are two wonderful ways to reduce your stress and anxiety levels.

My favorite breathing exercise is the 4-7-8 breath. Dr. Andrew Weil was one of my lecturers in school, and I remember him stating something to the effect of, "If you don't remember anything else I tell you today, remember this breathing exercise." I have used this exercise with numerous clients and have been told that it has helped tremendously with their sleep and anxiety. One of my clients said she can't even get through the whole series without falling asleep.

The technique is really quite simple. First, you breathe out all of the air in your lungs through your mouth. Next, breathe in for a count of four through your nose, with your tongue placed behind your front teeth. Hold the breath for a count of seven. Breathe out through your mouth for a count of eight. Do four sets of these at each sitting. The first few times you may feel a bit dizzy. This is normal. You should do this at least two times per day, once in the morning and once just before bed. The effects are cumulative. You should begin to feel more relaxed. You can also use this method occasionally during the day if you are feeling especially anxious or stressed.

Meditation is a fantastic stress reliever. There are both physical and mental benefits to using meditation:

Physical Benefits: Meditation reduces blood pressure, improves energy levels, reduces the risk of heart disease and stroke. Mindfulness practice helps to decrease inflammation and chronic conditions. Meditation can also reduce the risk of Alzheimer's disease and pre-mature death. More importantly for you, meditation also helps to treat menopausal symptoms! The fact remains that menopause stress can make us old! It can contribute to osteoporosis, the loss of skin elasticity, memory loss, and weight gain. By calming your mind and heart, you can reduce those menopausal symptoms and find some happiness! Meditation will most definitely help you get your *happy* back!

Mental Benefits: Meditation decreases anxiety and emotional instability, improves your mood, helps with rapid memory recall, improves learning, and can even help with ADD. For many of us menopausal women, we find that multitasking adds another layer of stress to our lives that we just don't need at this stage of the game. Meditation can help us from falling into that multitasking trap. You will gain the focus to stay on certain tasks longer, switching tasks less frequently.

There are many ways for you to begin a meditation routine. Do a search for meditation instructors in your area. You can also find many websites with self-guided instruction. There are wonderful meditation apps that you can download to your phone. One that I like to recommend to my clients is *Stop, Breathe, Think.* This app was created by Tools for Peace and is free! I love the descriptions of each command: Stop: Stop what you are doing. Check in with what you are thinking and how you are feeling. Breathe: Practice mindful breathing to create space between your thoughts, emotions, and reactions. Think: Learn to broaden your perspective and strengthen your force field of peace and calm by practicing one of the meditations.

Meditation may be one of the best and most effective things that you can do to relieve stress and anxiety in your life while providing you with a sense of calm and happiness.

Let's be frank. It is easier to pop a pill, especially one that promises to ease your symptoms as simple as 1-2-3. As with anything in the big pharma world—diet, anxiety, depression, weight loss, etc.—they tout the benefits of "ease" and simplicity! Take this pill, feel better. Whether it is hot flashes, diet, depression, anxiety, or even IBS, if you don't get to the cause of your symptoms and address them, you've fixed nothing. You are masking the reasons for your symptoms. The side effects of the drugs that are continuously prescribed to menopausal women, or even women in general, wreak havoc on our bodies.

Numerous clients who I have coached were prescribed anti-depressants and anti-anxiety drugs for hot flashes. They tell me that they do help with the hot flashes, but at what cost? They've also said that they didn't like the way the drugs made them feel. The side effects of taking these drugs could cause other health issues. The problem lay within the "healthcare industry." Doctors normally don't study holistic approaches to healthcare. What we really have is a "disease management industry." Possibly, a holistic method could be the first course of action for menopausal symptoms. Hiring a knowledgeable health coach could be quite beneficial to women in this phase of life. You won't find true happiness in a pill. You will probably find happiness, however, through your sheer will.

Obviously, my anxiety was brought on by my inability to deal with the loss of my dear friend. Often, women with mild anxiety or no previous symptoms of anxiety find that during the menopausal years, hormone imbalances and the perception of feeling as if they are "aging" can contribute to the onset of anxiety and depression. No anxiety or depression drug was going to "cure" me of my hurt and the physical symptoms that manifested themselves in my grieving mind and body. They may ease the symptoms in the short term, but forever? I think not. However, a combination of several holistic, healthy alternatives just might, and in my case, did.

I want you to concentrate on changing your mindset. You can't live a positive life with a negative mind. You must really believe that you can fix this! You must surround yourself with positive influences. These include people who lift you up, books and audio which inspire you (look for some suggestions in my resource guide), as well as activities that bring you joy and fulfillment. You are a woman who is strong. You are a woman who can overcome what life throws at her.

You'll need to do some good work. You'll need to do some extensive self-care, but believe me, it's worth it! You are worth it!

You can overcome your anxiety and depression! You can get your *happy* back!

CREATING MAGICAL MOMENTS

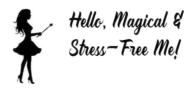

Hello, Magical &
Stress-Free Me!

What can I reduce to alleviate my stress and anxiety? Check off all that apply. Create a plan on how to eliminate each item.

_____ Caffeine

_____ Wine/Alcohol

_____ Excessive News

_____ Violent Media

_____ Computer/Device Time

What positive things can I do to help alleviate my stress and anxiety? Create an action plan and put it in motion.

- Counseling

- Gratitude journaling

- Breathing exercises: the 4-7-8 Breath

- Meditation: use the Stop Breath Think app

- Try some supplements (check with your doctor first): vitamin B complex, fish oil, magnesium, L-theanine, probiotic, and probiotic foods.

- Drink herbal teas

GRATITUDE JOURNAL

_____

_____

_____

_____

_____

_____

_____

_____

_____

_____

_____

_____

_____

_____

_____

_____

_____

_____

_____

_____

_____

_____

_____

_____

_____

_____

_____

_____

_____

_____

_____

_____

_____

_____

_____

_____

_____

_____

_____

_____

_____

_____

_____

_____

_____

_____

_____

_____

_____

THREE

Hot Stuff!!
And Other Body Plagues!

The covers are on, the covers are off, the covers are on, the covers are off. One leg juts out from beneath the covers to help cool your toasty body. Thirty seconds later, a chill sends you back cuddling under those protective layers. Your significant other is wondering what the heck all the flapping and sighing going on is. Then, once the hot flashes and night sweats awaken you, your brain decides now is not a good time to go back into REM mode. Instead, it decides it is time to create lists and tasks, and to recount yesterday's mishaps, or even those from ten years ago. Or, it might be considering what to make for dinner for the company you're having next week, or even on September 15th, 2040. Well, maybe not that specific, but actually, yes, sometimes that specific. Then, once you are awake and your mind takes over, it is time for that evil monster, ANXIETY, to pay a visit. You find it impossible to turn off your mind. Your body seems to have become your own worst enemy. It is not playing by the rules. It is not following the rules of engagement. It is time to SLAY THE ENEMY!!

We often find ourselves with financial woes, relationship issues, working too many hours, the inability to sleep, a poor or inconvenient diet, too many responsibilities, worrying about our kids, our parents, and life in general! What is happening and how do we fix it??

The organs and glands in our female bodies that control most of our hormones are the thyroid, adrenals, ovaries, pituitary, and pancreas. Our gut also plays a big part in our hormone balance. If you have an unhealthy or leaky gut, chances are, it is affecting your hormone balance.

Women often find that menopause is an extremely stressful time. This is often due to the hormone imbalances, lack of sleep, hot flashes, and other symptoms, along with the demands of life at this time. Quite often, the stress of caring for an aging parent or teenage children, along with a spouse who may be experiencing a mid-life crisis can all coincide at this time of your life. Feeling overwhelmed is most definitely an understatement.

Quite possibly, as a menopausal woman, you may be suffering from adrenal fatigue. This is a common condition and often debilitating symptom of menopause. Our adrenal glands are two small glands that sit just above the kidneys and are part of our endocrine system. They produce the hormones we need, especially in times of stress. Your symptoms of adrenal fatigue may differ from someone else's. The most common symptoms include feeling overly tired in the morning, even after a good night's sleep, the inability to handle stress, fatigue throughout the day, a weakened immune system, cravings for salty foods, and a higher energy level in the evenings. Other symptoms that may be linked to the ones already mentioned are weight gain, dark circles under the eyes, poor circulation, low blood sugar, low blood pressure, loss of muscle tone, joint pain, frequent urination, dry skin, dizziness, and allergies or respiratory ailments.

There are both physical and psychological causes for this disorder. The psychological cause is due to the adrenal glands' inability to deal with anxiety and stress. Normally, the adrenal glands organize the body's response to stress through hormones that control heart rate, immune function, energy production, and more. When there is an inability to meet the demands of daily stress, then there will be imbalances in body functions as well as emotional instability, leading to adrenal fatigue during menopause. The physical causes are triggered through the decrease in estrogen levels. Estrogen regulates the level of cortisol, which becomes uncontrolled when estrogen levels drop, in turn, causing adrenal fatigue. Maintaining hormone balance during menopause is of the utmost importance in preventing adrenal fatigue.

Our hormones play a significant role in keeping our bodies running like a well-oiled machine. They are like little soldiers, standing guard and stepping in when we find ourselves falling prey to some sort of internal battle being waged within our borders. If they are not kept balanced and in tune, in much the same way as an army is kept well trained, we find ourselves feeling threatened and "attacked." This modus operandi could be those sudden hot flashes or night sweats. It could be the inability to lose weight or bouts of anxiety. It could be a lack of energy, bad skin, or even severe cravings. So which hormones are responsible for our peaceful wellbeing? Here is a list of the brave soldiers and their tasks of keeping you well protected and at peace:

- Cortisol is an important hormone that is secreted by the adrenal glands. It is commonly known as the "stress hormone," as it plays a major role in the body's fight-or-flight response.

It is also involved in regulating blood pressure, blood sugar (glucose) levels, anti-inflammatory actions, and central nervous system activation. The body releases cortisol when it feels threatened or is under stress. In the days of early man, such an episode may have been a brief event, like fleeing an attacking animal or some other abrupt threat. The problem today is that these stressful events come more in the way of a continuous threat, such as work or school issues. Quite often, relationship and financial problems lead to prolonged stress. There are so many daily events that contribute to our stress levels staying elevated for an extended period of time, leading to chronic stress. When we find ourselves in this stressed state, the body keeps producing cortisol, keeping the levels high in our bodies. This leads to negative health effects like weight gain, heart disease, anxiety, and digestive problems.

- DHEA (Dehydroepiandrosterone) is a hormone that comes from the adrenal gland and is also made in the brain. DHEA leads to the production of the male and female sex hormones, androgen and estrogen. The levels of this hormone decrease with age, and more quickly in women. According to the Mayo Clinic, "Lower DHEA levels are found in people with hormonal disorders, HIV/AIDS, Alzheimer's disease, heart disease, depression, diabetes, inflammation, immune disorders, and osteoporosis. Corticosteroids, birth control taken by mouth, and agents that treat psychiatric disorders may reduce DHEA levels."

- Adrenaline, the fight-or-flight hormone, is also called epinephrine. This hormone is crucial to the body's response to a perceived threat or danger. However, overexposure to this hormone can be very detrimental to your health and well-being. Often times, adrenaline may be released when we are really not under any serious threat or danger. When this hormone is released in excess it can lead to a jittery, nervous feeling, insomnia, and even heart damage.

- Estrogen & progesterone are our sex hormones. First, let's look at estrogen. This is the hormone responsible for female physical features and reproduction. It will help to protect your bone health, will keep cholesterol in control as well as affects your brain and moods, heart, and skin. The ovaries produce most of the estrogen in your body. The adrenals make small amounts. Estrogen travels through your blood and affects your entire body. Too much estrogen can lead to health issues in women. These include weight gain mainly in your hips, waist and thighs, bad PMS, either a heavy or too light menstrual cycle, low libido, fibroids, fibrocystic breasts, fatigue, anxiety, and depression. Too little estrogen, most commonly caused by menopause or removal of the ovaries, can lead to a different set of problems including hot flashes, a dry vagina, trouble sleeping, dry skin, and mood swings. Estrogen levels can drop by 40-60% at menopause. I would regularly get a migraine headache when my estrogen levels dropped right before my period, especially when I was perimenopausal.

Progesterone prepares the endometrium (inner mucus membrane of the uterus) for a potential pregnancy after ovulation. During menopause, a woman's progesterone levels can drop much lower than her estrogen levels, upsetting the natural balance of these two hormones. By post menopause, levels of progesterone may reach 0%. One of the most well-known roles that this hormone plays in the body is its ability to oppose the cancer causing effect of estrogen on the endometrium. For this reason, it is often included in hormone replacement therapy (HRT) for women who have not had a hysterectomy. It can also help to slow the digestive process, build and maintain healthy bones, reduce anxiety, and increase sleepiness. Be aware that low progesterone levels can also lead to higher estrogen levels, which in effect, can decrease sex drive, contribute to weight gain, or cause gallbladder problems.

MENOPAUSE MOMENTS

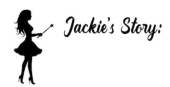 *Jackie's Story:*

"Menopause started showing up in my forties. I was working for a printing company at the time. While working, I'd feel a rush of heat take over me, starting at my toes and rising slowly up to my head, just like in the old cartoons. It would occur sporadically. You can take blood tests to see if you're in menopause, but mine kept coming back negative. Then it just stopped. A few years later, it started again after I had started my own business painting murals and decorative painting. I was in the paint store where I always get my supplies. All of a sudden, I was so hot all over—not the rushing from toes to head kind, just an all over slow melt down. I was red and glistening. I asked the guys at the desk, "Is it hot in here?" and their bug eyes looked at each other, saying, *no, no it isn't hot in here,* like they knew before I did that I was flashing. That was my first experience with that kind of heat sensation.

I found myself lacking patience, which I truly had plenty of most of the time, until I'd get my period. My husband was always using that as an excuse for my lack of patience during those weeks. I'd re-mind him, to no avail, that I have less of it when I'm crampy! Not to mention, if you knew my husband, well, that's a whole other story... I remember being in the kitchen and he said something to me and I just went off on him in one nasty sentence. Immediately, I was shocked at what just came out of my mouth. Did I just say that? Even I heard myself bark that time! I knew this had to be the beginning. Then the flashing began all the time, all day long, intermittently. It felt like someone turned on a heat lamp over me and followed me around. I'd be red and glistening. There was no *off* button. No escape. I just had to ride it out. Mind over matter.... or in the dead of winter, stand outside without a coat and feel relief.

At night, it was hard to fall asleep. It seemed I'd flash every time I laid down. I never had the drenching in the nighttime that I'd heard of. I just drank lots of water and had to make many bathroom runs during the night. When my husband was in the mood to cuddle, I'd try to talk myself into relaxing, knowing I was going to overheat at any moment, and sure enough, I'd rip the covers off. I'd break out into a sweat, and when he saw me start to glisten, he'd retreat. For the first time, I was laying outside of the sheets, in the cold, and he was freezing under the covers! I used to wear socks and nightgowns to bed! I couldn't imagine what summer would be like.

Summer ended up not being that bad. By then, I was used to overheating. I now understood why this woman kept blowing air out of her mouth while shopping at Marshalls. I kept looking at her. What is wrong with you? But now, I get it! It's kind of like child birth. The breathing technique helps you get through it. I finally finished a full year without a period. Menopause complete! The flashes are fewer but still can be as intense. I've started keeping a pretty fan in my pocket book. I don't care who sees me fanning myself. It feels good."

————

Jackie was diagnosed with uterine cancer shortly after she sent me her story in 2010. After chemotherapy and radiation, she is cancer free. She is trying to live a healthier lifestyle by eliminating sugar and processed foods and has added tai chi to her exercise routine. At the age of sixty-one, she has actually become an instructor.

MENOPAUSE MOMENTS

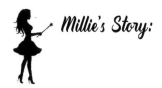 *Millie's Story:*

"I have many friends that are, like me, survivors and co-survivors of breast cancer, and we call ourselves 'breast friends.' Well, a few years ago, my breast friends and I decided to attend a Susan G. Komen Race for the Cure event in the foothills. For many years, I have been having hot flashes (now known as 'power surges'). I was on a medication called Tamoxifen to help fight off the cancer, but one of the side effects is hot flashes. The flashes got so bad that they would actually fog up my eyeglasses, and fourteen years later, they still do. During that weekend, my breast friends and I shared a hotel room. There were four of us. My hot flashes were so bad that I just couldn't get to sleep, so I finally got out of bed and took my pillow and slept on top of the air conditioner unit for the rest of the night. To this day, the girls still laugh about it."

———

Jackie and Millie are just two of the millions of women out there dealing with the uncomfortable symptoms of menopause. We can laugh about it, but we don't have to live with it! It doesn't have to be so.

So how do we fight back and get our hormones in balance, thus keeping all of those negative health issues at bay? Bring in the cavalry! Help is on the way!

As you prepare yourself to get in balance, there are certain things you should avoid as well as add to your lifestyle. As you do this, you may be resistant to giving up certain things, especially if you find yourself craving them. As you begin to change your mindset, keep this quote in the back of your mind: "Nothing tastes as good as healthy feels." You will be so thankful you listened to your body rather than your cravings.

Things to avoid while trying to get your hormones in balance or while addressing your adrenal fatigue include caffeine, alcohol, all sugars, refined grains, processed foods, fruit juices, gluten, artificial sweeteners, bacon and other processed meats. What effect do these play on your hormone imbalances? Let's start with caffeine. There are continuing studies being done on the link between caffeine and its effect on female hormones. The results are still a bit confusing. One thing they all agree on is that caffeine does effect estrogen levels, whether it lowers or increases levels is based not only on the amount of consumption, but on race and age as well. At this point, you are better off just eliminating it for the sake of balancing your hormones. You may want to note that caffeine does trigger hot flashes and anxiety as well. Maybe just kick those roasted beans to the wayside for now.

So what about alcohol? I am often amused when I begin coaching a woman who is either perimenopausal or menopausal because when we talk about what they are consuming, quite frequently, the first thing they will tell me is, "Don't make me give up my wine!" Inevitably, once they reduce or eliminate the wine, they are amazed at how much better they feel! They have reduced cravings, sleep well, and have an overall better sense of wellbeing. There are so many ways in which alcohol effects women's health in general, from the time they are adolescents all the way through menopause. For the purpose of this book, we will focus on how alcohol effects women during and after menopause. As it is high in calories and low in nutritional value, alcohol often contributes to weight gain in menopausal women. Some of the other negative effects of drinking alcohol include an increased risk of heart disease, stroke, high blood pressure, as well as breast cancer in women who are going through menopause.

Consuming alcohol also interferes with calcium absorption, which is a nutrient so important in maintaining bone density as well as other bodily functions. The amount of alcohol you consume also makes a difference in its effect on your health. The American Cancer Society warns that alcohol is linked to an increased risk of developing breast cancer, and that risk increases with the amount of alcohol consumed. Additional research shows a strong relationship between alcohol consumption and developing certain cancers, including mouth, liver, and esophageal cancer. There is continuing research on how alcohol affects hormone levels. At this time, it is best to limit or eliminate your alcohol consumption for your best health.

Got a sweet tooth? Let's take a look at how those refined sugars are affecting your hormone balance. You might want to keep a food diary for a week or so to see just how your sugar intake effects your moods. You will most likely find that sugar contributes to extreme highs and lows in both your energy levels and your moods. It can also disrupt insulin, which is one of the most powerful hormones in your body. This hormone is connected to all of the other hormones in your body, including estrogen and testosterone. Because of this connection, sugar may be the main culprit that leads to many symptoms that can become worse during menopause such as hot flashes, night sweats, insomnia, anxiety, and irritability. Of course, realistically, you can't remove all sugar from your diet, nor should you have to. What you should do is limit your glycemic load by eliminating refined carbohydrates and consuming complex carbohydrates, healthy fats, protein, and fibers. Your body will say, "Thank you!"

You've been led to believe by the food industry that a healthy substitute for sugar is an artificial sweetener. This could not be further from the truth. When we eat or drink something sweet, two things happen. Your brain releases dopamine, activating its reward center. Leptin is also released. This is the appetite regulating hormone. Leptin sends a message to your brain that you are "full" when you have consumed a certain number of calories. Contrarily, when you are ingesting something that tastes sweet but doesn't have any calories, your brain's reward center is activated, but the calories never arrive, so there is nothing to de-activate it. Since the calories never come, your body will continue to signal that it needs more. In essence, artificial sweeteners are deceiving your body into thinking that calories are on the way! Your body keeps on thinking that it needs more. Guess what happens next? You crave carbs!!

As a menopausal woman, you probably are struggling enough with maintaining your weight. You don't need to include a crappy sugar substitute that can contribute to other health issues as well. Weight gain, insulin sensitivity, cardiovascular disease, stroke, and Alzheimer's disease are some of the health problems you might experience. These are the same issues you might encounter from excessive sugar consumption. So just how are these artificial sweeteners a "healthy" substitute? You are sweet enough darlin'! No fake stuff needed! If you need to add some "sweet" to your life, try using coconut sugar, maple syrup, or local honey. These are all low-glycemic alternatives, of course, in moderation.

You've heard all the hype about eating gluten-free. You can find gluten in foods that contain wheat, barley, rye, and some oats (look for oats specifically labeled "gluten-free"). Possibly, you think this is just the latest diet craze. For some, it is not a necessary diet. The fact, however, remains that statistics show about 1 in 133 people have celiac disease, which is an inherited autoimmune disease that causes damage to the small intestine when gluten is ingested. In turn, this prevents nutrients from being absorbed into the body. There is another .4% of people who have a doctor-diagnosed wheat allergy. Regarding an even larger group of people, according to The National Foundation for Celiac Awareness, "As many as 18 million Americans have some non-celiac sensitivity to gluten."

The symptoms of celiac disease are numerous and vary from person to person. In some adults with celiac disease, an inability to absorb calcium can lead to osteoporosis. Both of my daughters have celiac disease. My oldest daughter actually had osteopenia (decreased bone density) at the age of twenty, which was discovered upon her celiac diagnosis. My younger daughter is still struggling with anemia—another symptom which affects folks with the disease. The following is a list of common symptoms for adults with celiac disease:

- Iron deficiency

- Bone or joint pain

- Arthritis

- Depression or anxiety

- Bone loss or osteoporosis

- Tingling numbness in hands and feet

- Seizures

- Erratic menstrual periods

- Dermatitis herpetiformis

- Mouth sores

If you feel you may have celiac disease, DO NOT stop eating gluten until you have a true diagnosis. If you stop eating gluten and then go for testing, which is a simple blood panel, you may get a false negative result. If you do, indeed, have celiac disease, you will want a true diagnosis, as this could affect your medical insurance, as well as the possibility you may need further testing for other medical conditions attributed to the disease. It is of the utmost importance to be tested as soon as possible if you feel you may have the disease as to avoid possible long term effects such as malnutrition, liver disease, and in rare cases, cancers of the intestine.

You may not have celiac disease, but you may be gluten sensitive. Your symptoms may include bloating, diarrhea, constipation, gas, nausea, acid reflux, and intestinal cramping. It is important to note that up to sixty percent of irritable bowel syndrome (IBS) patients have been misdiagnosed. They may actually be gluten sensitive. About only twenty percent of folks that have gluten sensitivity suffer with gastrointestinal problems. The rest may be gluten sensitive without even realizing it. Since most people associate gluten sensitivity with digestive issues, they may not consider that gluten could be at the root of their health concerns. The following list of health conditions could stem from gluten sensitivity: depression, muscle and joint pain, fatigue, migraines, multiple sclerosis, fibromyalgia, chronic fatigue syndrome, psoriasis, eczema and other skin rashes, lupus, scleroderma, Sjogren's syndrome, asthma, dementia, ADD, ADHD, OCD, osteopenia, osteoporosis, diabetes, thyroid disease, cardiomyopathy, chronic anemia, coordination problems and anemia.

So, as a menopausal woman, just how could gluten be effecting you? It also can impact your hormones (endocrine system) as well as affect your adrenal glands by placing stress on them. By putting stress on your adrenals, they become exhausted and your bodily systems start to break down. They are unable to repair themselves. They slow down, which can lead to menopausal symptoms such as fatigue, depression, hot flashes, and low libido. When under chronic stress, the adrenals begin to produce stress hormones at the expense of your sex hormones, especially progesterone. There is evidence to suggest that taking gluten out of your diet may help to balance your hormones. What an easy way to see if something as simple as removing gluten from your diet could actually change everything about your life!

If you've been tested for celiac disease and the results are negative, there are saliva and stool tests that can be performed to see if you have a gluten sensitivity. These tests will pick up antibodies in your saliva or stool. Be aware that blood tests are not accurate in determining gluten intolerance/sensitivity. They are only useful for diagnosing full blown celiac disease. Another easy way to see if you might have gluten sensitivity is to remove gluten from your diet and keep a food journal. See how you feel. Give it some time. A sample journal is below. You can use this for any type of elimination diet, for example, if you want to try removing dairy or meat from your diet to see if your symptoms improve. There are many gluten-free items available now for those who need them. Some of my favorite flours are almond and coconut. Keep in mind that eating gluten-free, when it comes to processed and baked goods, does not necessarily mean "healthier." Many of these foods use rice flours which actually have a higher glycemic load. To truly eat a "healthy" gluten-free diet, stick to whole foods and try to keep away from the processed junk.

There are other ways that your diet and nutrition play a part in your hormone imbalance. There are known hormone disruptors in many of the foods we consume. As a baby boomer, I grew up eating processed lunch meats. Money was scarce so our usual lunches consisted of the cheapest meats available. My least favorite was olive loaf. YUCK!! Basically, this was good old bologna inserted with slices of green olives with pimento. Not sure how that was even invented, but my mom discovered it and we ate it religiously through my elementary school years. My lunch meats fluctuated between olive loaf, bologna, and turkey or chicken roll. I believe that the process of becoming a roll was taking already processed meat, grinding it up, and turning it into another form of science experiment. Deli meats are full of nitrates and chemicals. Studies have shown that nitrates could lead to thyroid hormone disruption. Research has also shown that by eating processed meats you have an increased risk of premature death. Enough said about this. Stay away from them.

Other items on the "don't" list to stay away from are oils high in omega-6 such as corn, cottonseed, peanut, soybean, canola, safflower, and sunflower. You should instead boost your omega-3 intake with foods like chia seeds, walnuts, wild-caught fish, and grass-fed animal products. You can also add supplements that contain a type of omega-6 fat called GLA (Gamma-Linoleic Acid) like evening primrose oil, borage oil, or hemp seeds. Studies show that taking GLA can support healthy progesterone levels.

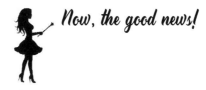 *Now, the good news!*

There are so many fantastic, delicious, and wonderful things you can still consume and enjoy! A well balanced whole food diet can help keep your hormones stable and balanced.

Things to do and include:

- Eat 3 meals per day. Make breakfast and lunch the larger meals, dinner should be light.

   Foods to include: organic fruits and vegetables, lean meats, poultry, fish, whole grains, beans, some dairy, nuts and seeds, healthy oils and fats. Drink lots of filtered water.

- Include 1-2 snacks per day. Make one at about 4pm, as this is often when energy levels are low.

- Eat protein at each meal, whether it is a lean meat, vegan, or vegetarian option. Beans are a great choice, but in moderation, as they can also be high in carbs. See how your body feels when consuming them. According to Dr. Christiane Northrup in *The Wisdom of Menopause*, "Protein needs vary depending upon your size and physical activity. The bigger and more active you are, the more you need. In general, if you have any tendency toward weight gain at midlife, your diet should be about forty percent protein, thirty-five percent low-glycemic index carbs, and twenty-five percent fat." She also states, "You don't have to adhere to this rigidly at every meal and snack, but it's an average to shoot for over about a week's time." (Northrup, 245)

- Pump up those organic green leafy fellas too! There are so many ways to incorporate more greens in your diet. Some options are:

    a. Breakfast: green smoothies or omelets.

    b. Lunch: big salads with a protein like chicken or tuna added, green smoothies, or sautéed veggies as a side.

    c. Dinner: side salad, sautéed or roasted greens as a side dish, added to soups.

Check out several easy recipes at the end of this chapter. You should try to include at least four to six helpings of greens daily. Leafy greens are full of vitamins, minerals, and disease fighting phytochemicals. If you do nothing else to change your lifestyle other than add a substantial amount of healthy greens, you'll be amazed at how well you will feel. More energy, less inflammation, and better skin, as well as boosting bone and eye health are just some of the fantastic benefits. Greens are also full of fiber, which can keep you feeling fuller longer, thus contributing to weight loss. Fiber can also lower cholesterol and blood pressure, along with keeping blood sugar levels stable. The benefits of consuming dark leafy greens are numerous and almost miraculous. For example, they also strengthen the immune system, prevent cancers, improve blood circulation, and so much more. Your body will be jumping for joy and thanking you for pumping up the greens! Some of your best buddies are kale, collards, Swiss chard, turnip greens, mustard greens, spinach, broccoli, red and green romaine lettuce, and cabbages.

- Eat a variety of healthy fats. Your body needs these for hormone production. They will also help you to boost your metabolism and lose weight. Some foods which contain these healthy buddies are avocados, wild-caught salmon, coconut oil, and grass-fed butter.

- Take your supplements! Along with the ones I've already mentioned, include a daily vitamin D3. Vitamin D deficiency is extremely detrimental to your health! Studies show that two-thirds of women are vitamin D deficient. What might be causing this deficiency? Possibly a lack of sun exposure, omega-3 fat balance, skin color, or even your location can influence your vitamin D levels. Did you know it can help to prevent breast cancer? Seventy percent of women who are diagnosed with breast cancer are vitamin D deficient. Vitamin D has been shown to prevent breast cancer cell growth. Breast cancer risk is reduced when your D levels reach 40 ng/ml. Supplementing with around 2,000 IU/daily can reduce an incidence of breast cancer by fifty percent. Our risk of developing cancer, including breast cancer, increases with age. Ninety-five percent of women who develop breast cancer are over the age of forty, thus the importance of supplementing with D3 for menopausal women. Also, some drugs used to manage menopausal symptoms may either increase or decrease a woman's cancer risk.

Another fantastic reason to take your D is for healthy bones! Women who are D deficient are seventy-seven percent more likely to suffer a hip fracture, and giving elderly women vitamin D has been shown to increase life expectancy by two years. Weak and brittle bones do not have to be an unavoidable consequence of aging! The vitamin D counsel recommends you take a minimum of 1000 IU per twenty-five pounds of body weight. The time is now to become a D3 diva!

- Other beneficial supplements that can help with balancing your hormones are adaptogen herbs. These herbs are natural healers that improve your body's ability to resist multiple forms of stress. They also work to balance your hormones while protecting your body from a whole list of diseases. These herbs include ashwagandha and holy basil. Each of these has been shown to boost immune function, combat stress, lower cholesterol, protect cardiovascular health, improve thyroid function, stabilize blood sugar, enhance energy, and reduce anxiety and depression.

More herbs that help with menopausal symptoms:

- Black cohosh: This herb has been used for generations by women all over the world. Many of my clients use this for their hot flashes.

- Red clover: This herb is rich in phytoestrogens.

- Chastetree: Recent studies show that properties of this herb may mimic the soothing actions of progesterone.

- Kudzu: This herb is a member of the pea family and is native to Asia. Much like red clover, it contains phytochemicals that function in a protective fashion.

- Passionflower: This herb has antidepressant and anti-anxiety properties.

- Pueraria Mirifica: This is a plant that women in southeast Asia have been using for over seven hundred years to relieve menopausal symptoms such as hot flashes and night sweats, as well as promote a restful sleep, stabilize mood, and contribute to smoother skin. I have been using this supplement for about six months at the time of this writing and have experienced fewer hot flashes and a reduction in the severity of my migraines. The specific supplement I take is A-ma-ta, which was created by Dr. Christiane Northrup. I recommended A-ma-ta to my younger sister, who was suffering with severe hot flashes, and within a week, they disappeared.

- Wild yam: This herb can be used for both menopause and menstrual related symptoms.

Add some potent antioxidants as well! These will help you fight the good fight with those free radicals that can cause all kinds of damage and disease in your body from macular degeneration and cataracts to heart disease and cancer. Eating a rainbow of colors with your veggies and fruits is a great place to start. You can pump up your antioxidants through supplements as well. Some of my favorites are Pycnogenol, Resveratrol, and Ubiquinol. Pycnogenol French maritime pine bark extract acts as a potent blend of antioxidants. It is a natural anti-inflammatory, stimulates generation of collagen and hyaluronic acid, and helps with natural dilation of blood vessels by supporting the production of nitric oxide. It has multiple anti-aging benefits too. Resveratrol is a supplement made from red wine or red grape extracts. Research suggests that this supplement is also beneficial in protecting the body from heart disease, cancer, diabetes, and Alzheimer's. According to research, the body is protected from the harmful effects of these and other age related diseases due to Resveratrol's ability to activate the SIRT1 gene, which is a biological mechanism that protects the body. Ubiquinol (this is the reduced, active, and more absorbable antioxidant form of CoQ10) is the "antioxidant that actually restores all your other antioxidants. The critical 'spark' that keeps your heart beating strong. Without a doubt, it's one of the most remarkable discoveries of the 21st century. Put simply: This amazing nutrient is the 'energy switch' that sparks life to all 100 trillion cells in your body." See my Resource Guide for recommendations for these three supplements.

By following a healthy whole food diet, you should experience a tremendous difference in your menopausal symptoms. You should have less hot flashes, more energy, more restful sleep, better concentration, and feel more positive in your moods.

There may be hormone disruptors lurking around your home in the form of personal care items and kitchen tools. By changing them, you can greatly help to eliminate toxins in your body which might be contributing to hormone disruption. Do not use body care products that are high in parabens, propylene glycol, sodium lauryl sulfate and DEA. Stay away from Teflon pans and try using stainless steel, ceramic, or cast iron for cooking. Replace plastic bottles with glass or stainless steel to reduce the toxic effects of BPA (BisPhenol A), an industrial chemical which has been found to leach into food and beverages.

Another possible hormone disrupting culprit is birth control pills. Birth control raises estrogen to potentially dangerous levels and can lead to an increased risk of breast cancer, blood clotting, heart attack, and stroke. They may also cause migraines, mood changes, increased blood pressure, gallbladder disease, nausea, irregular bleeding or spotting, and weight gain. You may want to experiment instead with some phytoestrogens or adaptogen herbs listed previously in this chapter.

Do your due diligence when investigating the possibility of using phytoestrogens. Excessive use of them may potentially stimulate breast cancer growth as well as increase the risk of cognitive decline and dementia. Phytoestrogens are complicated. If you feel phytoestrogens could help you, please check with your healthcare provider first to see if taking a phytoestrogen is safe for you.

Your body may also be craving exercise! As we move on in years, somehow, the majority of women tend to move around a lot less! This is why osteoporosis has reached epidemic levels in the U.S. We need to be doing more for our bodies! We especially need to concentrate on weight bearing exercises to help build strong bones. It is lack of exercise, not the number of candles on your birthday cake, that determines what condition your body is in. You've got to use those muscles! Remember the old saying, "Use it or lose it!" Well, repeat daily to condition your mind so that you can concentrate on ways to condition your body!

Now, I am not advocating a strenuous routine like CrossFit, running marathons, or participating in triathlons (that is, unless, you wish to and are capable of doing it!). I am suggesting, however, that you find something doable. Something you can put on your calendar at least three to four times a week that gets your heart pumping and your body working. This can be as simple as a brisk thirty to forty-five-minute walk, yoga, Pilates, tai chi, or a recent pleasure of mine, rebounding. A rebounder is a small trampoline that you can easily store in your home. NASA has deemed it more effective than a treadmill. This is quite beneficial for your legs and feet as there is less pressure, thus less foot and leg pain. Rebounding is also fantastic for your lymphatic system as it boosts drainage and immune function. Rebounding can improve your digestion, is great for your skeletal system and increasing bone mass, is more than two times as effective as running with no knee or ankle stress, increases endurance on a cellular level by stimulating mitochondrial production (responsible for cell energy), helps to circulate oxygen throughout your body, improves balance, helps improve the effects of other exercise, and some sources claim that rebounding can help support the thyroid and adrenals. It is a whole body exercise that is beneficial for muscle tone throughout your body.

There are numerous benefits to exercising including weight control, fighting health conditions and disease, it gives you an energy boost, improves your sleep, boosts your libido, and improves your mood! If you want to balance those hormones, short high intensity exercise has been shown to help, especially in folks over forty. Exercise stimulates various brain chemicals, so taking a brisk walk or getting in a quick workout will do wonders to help you get your happy back!

If you want to stay healthy, you'll need to concentrate on getting at least thirty minutes of exercise in per day. You'll need to pump it up a bit more for weight loss. See how you feel. Everyone is different. Experiment with different types of exercise to see what best suits your likes and needs. Don't be afraid to try new things! Maybe a dance or swim class? Possibly belly dancing or even pole dancing? Get adventurous! Have fun!

Find what works for you and your body, and make it a habit that is sustainable as well as enjoyable. Of course, the more often you do this, the healthier and happier you will become!

So you've pumped up the exercise, why is your body still feeling stressed or out of balance? Probably because you are skipping some good ZZZ's. This is probably one of the most abused hormone disrupters. You have permission to sleep more! That's right! For the sake of your hormone balance, you must get at least seven to eight hours of sleep each night. Did you know that your hormones are on a schedule? Cortisol, the stress hormone, is regulated at midnight. So if you are getting to bed too late, your body is not getting a break from the sympathetic fight-or-flight stress response. It's no wonder that there are so many stress related disorders now. Ideally, you should be in bed by 10pm. Your best sleep is between 10pm and 2am, as endocrinologists (hormone experts) claim that one hour of sleep between those times is equal to two hours of sleep either before or after those times.

There you go! Some easy steps to get you back to your happy, healthy self. Start putting them in action today. It is never too soon to get your life in balance!

I can guarantee that by following a healthy whole food diet, taking your supplements, exercising as described above, getting some good sleep, along with eliminating those environmental nasties that can throw your hormones out of balance you will experience a tremendous difference in your menopausal symptoms. You should have less hot flashes, more energy, restful sleep, better concentration, and feel more positive in your moods. Your serotonin and endorphin levels will be partying like crazy. You'll most definitely be getting your *happy* back!

MAGICAL GREEN RECIPES

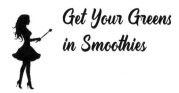

Get Your Greens in Smoothies

Use this as a basic plan for your smoothies!

Makes two helpings! One for now, one for later (or one to share)!

Pick one from each column and add them to your high speed blender in this order, then blend them all up for a healthy daily treat!

LIQUIDS: (2 cups)

- Water
- Coconut milk
- Coconut water
- Almond milk
- Kefir

GREENS: (2 cups)

- Spinach
- Kale
- Swiss chard
- Dandelion greens
- Romaine
- (If you like a little kick, add a bit of arugula!)

FRUIT: (3 cups: mix them up!) Use some frozen fruit to make your magical concoction nice and chilled!

- Pineapple
- Blueberries
- Raspberries
- Strawberries
- Blackberries
- Banana
- Peach
- Apple
- Avocado
- Orange
- Acai berries (great antioxidant)

BOOSTERS: Just give it a sprinkle!

- Chia seeds
- Flax seeds
- Hemp seeds
- Cacao nibs (chocolatey goodness!)
- Maca root powder: This may help with that libido and enhance your mood!
- Spirulina: An amazing superfood rich in protein, vitamins, minerals, carotenoids and antioxidants, this blue-green algae is also a great antioxidant that fights off free radicals. It is also rich in beta-carotene so it may fight cancer and act as a great anti-aging supplement. It is known to lower blood pressure, decrease bad cholesterol, increase stamina, build lean muscle mass, and give your system a natural cleanse! To top it all off, it is a complete protein!
- Matcha powder (powdered green tea): Made from high quality

tea, you are consuming the actual leaves. This makes it more nutritionally potent than if you steeped the tea leaves. It is very high in antioxidants. It does contain caffeine, but usually provides you with an "alert" calmness, as it contains the natural substance, L-Theanine (which I talked about earlier). Don't drink it too close to bedtime!

Goodly Green Salad Dressings:

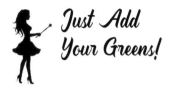

Just Add Your Greens!

ASIAN DELIGHT:

Ingredients:

¼ cup rice vinegar

2 tablespoons tamari

Juice of one orange

1 clove garlic, minced

1 tablespoon toasted sesame oil

1 tablespoon honey

1 teaspoon ginger, freshly grated

Directions:

Whisk all ingredients together in a bowl. Pour into a mason jar and refrigerate. Will stay for about one week.

GARLICKY GREENS DRESSING:

Ingredients:
¼ cup olive oil
2/3 cup red wine vinegar
2 garlic cloves, peeled and mashed
¼ teaspoon mustard powder
¼ teaspoon onion powder
Pinch of salt and pepper
1 teaspoon nutritional yeast (gives it a cheesy flavor, but dairy-free!)

Directions:
Put all ingredients in a jar and mix well! Store in refrigerator.

RASPBERRY VINAIGRETTE:

Ingredients:
1 cup raspberries (preferably organic!)
2 tablespoons honey
¼ cup olive or grapeseed oil
2/3 cup balsamic vinegar
Pinch of salt
Optional: Poppy Seeds

Directions:
Give the raspberries a swirl in a food processor. Add the honey, oil, vinegar, and salt. Pour into a mason jar and shake well. Store in refrigerator.

VEGETABLES: (CUT INTO BITE-SIZED PIECES)

Roasted: Pick a bunch and mix 'em up! You can roast just about any veggie! This is my absolute favorite way to eat my veggies! Your family will love them too!

Ingredients:

Cauliflower
Broccoli
Brussels sprouts
Bell peppers
Onions
Any type of root veggie: potatoes, sweet potatoes, parsnips, carrots

Directions:

Toss your veggies with a good amount of olive oil, coconut oil, or avocado oil.

Season them with salt and pepper to taste.

Pre-heat oven to 425°F.

Spread your veggies out on a baking sheet in a single layer, giving them plenty of room to roast! Use two sheets if you need to!

Roast until they are tender and toasty! You want them well cooked! Should take about 15-20 minutes. (Check at 15 minutes.)

When ready, toss with some fresh chopped herbs (tarragon, dill, mint, basil, parsley) if you like!

HINT: Some veggies take longer to cook then others (i.e.: cauliflower and broccoli). You can cook them separately or add onto baking sheet in stages. Cook the hardest veggies first, adding softer veggies later.

You can steam or sauté your veggies as well!

For steaming, if you don't have a steamer pot, you can improvise by just adding some water to your veggies in a pot with a matching lid.

For sautéing (a method of cooking food that uses a small amount of oil in a shallow pan over relatively high heat), you can either add some olive oil to the pan and cook (add a little crushed garlic, salt, and pepper for nice flavor!), or you can sauté in water as well.

CREATING MAGICAL MOMENTS

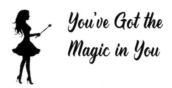

You've Got the Magic in You

You will want to begin working on balancing those hormones! A great start is to create magical healthy meals. Make a seven-day menu based on the suggestions in this chapter.

The best way to remember to get those greens in is to use the 1-2-3 Rule: 1 veggie for breakfast, 2 for lunch, and 3 for dinner (this can include a salad with several different veggies in it).

Use the following page to create your meal plans in the weeks ahead. Feel free to make copies and start planning ahead.

MENU PLANNING

	Breakfast	Snack	Lunch	Snack	Dinner	Beverage
Monday						
Tuesday						
Wednesday						
Thursday						
Friday						
Saturday						
Sunday						

GRATITUDE JOURNAL

_____

_____

_____

_____

_____

_____

_____

_____

_____

_____

_____

_____

_____

_____

_____

_____

_____

_____

_____

_____

_____

_____

_____

_____

_____

_____

_____

_____

_____

_____

_____

_____

_____

_____

_____

_____

_____

_____

_____

_____

_____

_____

_____

_____

_____

_____

_____

FOUR

Filling the Void: Life After Hysterectomy

So you've been told that you may be in need of a hysterectomy. Did you know that the word "hysterectomy" comes from the word "hysteria?" Indeed, many moons ago, hysterectomies were performed on women who showed signs of "hysteria." What we know now is that these symptoms were most likely anxiety and depression. A hysterectomy is an operation performed to remove the uterus. It can also include the removal of some or all of the other reproductive organs, including the ovaries. Nowadays, hysterectomies are just one of several options for women that are suffering from fibroids, severe menstrual cycles, endometriosis, cancer, or uterine prolapse (otherwise known as a dropped uterus). Such was the case for me.

Having delivered three very large babies vaginally (8lbs. 13 oz., 9lbs. 12 oz., and 10 lbs. 8 oz. YES!! 10½ lbs.!!! YIKES!!), my uterus was literally falling out of my body. Doesn't that present a lovely visual? Although I was not in any pain, it was a very uncomfortable feeling between my legs. On top of that, I was finding it hard to poop!

What also occurred in my precious baby producing vessel was what is known as a rectocele. This is when the end of the large intestine (rectum) pushes against the back wall of the vagina, moving it. At the time I had my hysterectomy, my urogynecologist performed a rectocele repair. Another badge of honor that may occur is what is known as an enterocele. This is when the small bowel presses against and moves the upper wall of the vagina. Rectoceles and enteroceles occur when the lower pelvic muscles are either damaged or weakened by labor, childbirth, aging, or previous pelvic surgeries. Although my rectocele occurred prior to my surgery for the hysterectomy, on occasion, either a rectocele, enterocele, or both can occur after a hysterectomy. How do you know if you have either of these 'celes? The usual symptoms include pain during intercourse or lower back pain. If you are concerned that you may have either a rectocele or enterocele, please see your gynecologist.

Before agreeing to the surgery, you should most definitely get a second opinion. Usually, a hysterectomy is recommended only after you've tried more conservative treatment options with no success. If you are suffering from any of these issues, you may want to explore non-surgical options first. For instance, to help with prolapse issues, there is a device known as a pessary. A pessary is a device worn inside the vagina which supports the bladder, vagina, or uterine apex, and rectum.

Many doctors today have realized that the uterus plays a role in regulating hormones. They don't advise having a hysterectomy unless it is completely necessary. In this regard, hysterectomies have become somewhat controversial. Check with your healthcare provider for all of your non-surgical options first.

If you do have a hysterectomy with oophorectomy, where your ovaries are being removed along with your uterus, then your body will go through what is described as "artificial menopause" or "surgically induced menopause." A hysterectomy can lead to sudden hormonal changes. Your doctor may prescribe estrogen replacement therapy or other types of meds to relieve your symptoms. Have a serious discussion with your physician about HRT therapy.

Although HRT can be effective in helping with menopausal symptoms, studies by the Women's Health Initiative involving mainly FDA approved PremPro, a combination of Premarin (conjugated equine estrogen) and Provera (medroxyprogesterone acetate), have led many to conclude that the risks of conventional HRT far outweigh the benefits for certain groups of women. The risks included coronary heart disease (CHD), invasive breast cancer, stroke, pulmonary embolism (PE), endometrial cancer, colorectal cancer, and hip fracture. If these synthetic hormones and meds cause too many side effects, you can ask your doctor about bio-identical or natural hormone replacement. Bio-identical hormones are those which are identical in molecular structure to the hormones that women make in their bodies. These hormones must be synthesized in a laboratory since, other than in a woman's body, these hormones are not found in nature. They are typically made from the extracts of soy or yams. Some FDA approved bio-identical hormones are available, while others can be compounded individually. Scientific studies have not found that using bio-identical HRT offers any health advantages over standard HRT.

If you care to go a more holistic route, many of the suggestions for balancing hormones throughout this book may be the best course of action for you. It doesn't hurt to begin holistically and avoid potentially uncomfortable side effects or health concerns from meds and artificial hormones. There is proof that for women over the age of fifty, phytoestrogens (plant based estrogens) can be beneficial. These benefits include a reduction in hot flashes, reduction in bone loss, and a boost in libido, while they also help to regulate iron absorption while possibly preventing or reducing certain types of cancers, enhancing heart health, and helping with weight loss. Some good phytoestrogen rich foods include lentils, oats, barley, sesame seeds, yams, alfalfa, apples, carrots, jasmine oil, wheat germ, tempeh, pomegranates, licorice root, red clover, and clary sage oil. Soy is often included in this list, however, I would suggest staying away from soy as a phytoestrogen supplement in high doses as there are studies to suggest it could be harmful. I would, however, encourage you to include traditional soy foods in your diet such as edamame, tempeh, miso, and soy sauce. Be sure that they are organic and non-GMO. Stay away from processed soy products and soy additives in foods.

If you have a thyroid condition, be sure to stay away from eating raw phytoestrogens, as goitrogens in these foods could interfere with thyroid function. Cooking them will prevent this, but do not consume within two hours of taking any thyroid medication.

A very good way to approach hormone balance from a holistic standpoint is to begin eating a mostly organic whole food diet prior to the procedure. You will want to make sure you are in good health physically as well as emotionally. Exercise regularly. Eliminate the nasties from your diet that could affect your hormone balance such as alcohol, caffeine, gluten, processed foods, and sugar. Reduce the chemicals in your environment. This includes your personal care and beauty items.

Look for brands that are organic and don't contain cancer causing or hormone disrupting (see propyl paraben) toxins. I personally love Sunshine Botanicals and Neal's Yard Remedies (NYR). Use the EWG (Environmental Working Group) app called Skin Deep to check out the items you have on hand.

MENOPAUSE MOMENTS

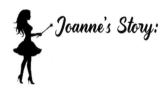

Joanne's Story:

A fellow health coach, Joanne, recently shared with me how she was experiencing hot flashes right after having a total hysterectomy. For months, the only thing she did was eat edamame (soy, a phytoestrogen) to see if it would help to reduce the occurrence of the flashes. They lessened, but did not disappear. Prior to her surgery, Joanne completed detox cleanses about four times a year. She hadn't done one in a while and recently decided to do a five-week detox. At the time of this writing, she has eliminated meats, dairy, gluten, caffeine, soy, and alcohol. Joanne has not experienced one hot flash! She will slowly add each back into her diet to see which one(s) may be triggering her "power surges." As I mentioned earlier, an elimination diet is a great way to figure out just what may be causing your symptoms. Check my Resource Guide for info on how to do it.

———

For me, the best course of action was to have the hysterectomy. I was extremely uncomfortable and having trouble having a bowel movement. At the time, and after discussing it with both my gynecologist and urogynecologist, I felt the surgery was what I needed. Since I had not gone through menopause yet, my doctor suggested I keep my ovaries. A woman's risk of ovarian cancer diminishes when her ovaries are removed, but the risks of dying from other more common causes rises, proving there is a benefit to the hormones ovaries provide. Since there was no history of ovarian cancer in my family, we both agreed that this would be a good choice for me.

I feel comfortable with my decision, but encourage those who are trying to decide what they should do to explore all options prior to agreeing to the surgical procedure. Surgery is serious business and carries with it risks and side effects. Be absolutely sure about your choices before going ahead with the procedure. This includes whether you are considering a total or partial (ovaries are left intact) hysterectomy.

Of course, continue your healthy lifestyle after your hysterectomy as well. By incorporating healthy daily habits, you are guaranteed to get those hormones in balance and live a longer, healthier, more comfortable, and *happier* life!

CREATING MAGICAL MOMENTS

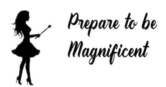

Prepare to be Magnificent

Could a hysterectomy be in your future? Creating a magical life begins with preparing your precious body to be at its utmost healthiest and happiest prior to the procedure.

Be sure to:

- Eat a healthy diet that includes lots of greens (as organic as possible)!

- Reduce environmental toxins (including self-care products).

- Exercise!

- Eliminate/reduce: wine/alcohol, caffeine, gluten, processed foods, and sugar.

Filling the Void: Life After Hysterectomy

GRATITUDE JOURNAL

_____

_____

_____

_____

_____

_____

_____

_____

_____

_____

_____

_____

_____

_____

_____

_____

_____

_____

_____

_____

_____

_____

FIVE

Sex & Sleep: Are You Getting Enough?

Sex and sleep—two extremely important, but often neglected events in our hectic lives. If a man was writing this, he might have said, "Two extremely important, *daily,* but often neglected events in our lives." You may be reading this and thinking, "Sex? Nah, I'm good. I wish he'd leave me alone and let me sleep!" Men and women are wired differently. In our stress filled lives, men often look to sex as a stress reliever, where women, on the other hand, need to be relaxed and stress-free to desire or enjoy sex. Women are two to three more times as likely to have a decrease in sex drive than men as they age. There are several factors that can lead to a woman's low libido. Hormone imbalances, which can cause unpleasant symptoms like hot flashes, night sweats, and vaginal dryness, may cause a woman to lose her desire and drive. The hormone, testosterone, which plays a part in women's sex drive and sensation, naturally decreases as we age.

Some, but not all, women who, upon undergoing an abrupt menopause in the case of the removal of both ovaries or by chemotherapy, may experience a greater reduction in their libido than women who experience a natural menopause. This is due to the immediate decrease of both estrogen and testosterone. Although known as the male sex hormone, testosterone is a natural female libido enhancer. It is made in the ovaries and adrenal glands. About fifty percent of testosterone is made in the ovaries, so once they are gone, poof! Half of your libido booster is gone! If you find that your libido has gone limp due to either of these events, try some of the holistic methods throughout this book to find hormonal nirvana. If you think you may need more help, ask your gynecologist about a bio-identical testosterone replacement.

The sad truth is, whatever the cause of your lack of interest, it can wreak havoc on the relationship with your significant other. So many jokes have been made about this particular subject, like women feigning headaches or faking an orgasm. When women meet in groups they talk and joke about their husbands' persistent nighttime requests and their own total disinterest in being a willing participant. A close friend of mine, I'll call her Nancy, relayed a story to me that had me in stitches. One day, she was in her car and talking on the phone with another mutual friend named Linda. As she was parked and talking to Linda, Nancy mentioned to her, "Today is a holy day of obligation." Now, as a Catholic, I know that this means that it is a day that you should be headed to church. So, with that in mind, Linda was a bit confused.

"Holy day of obligation? Am I forgetting something?"

Nancy laughed and said, "It's our wedding anniversary. A holy day of obligation, you know, the day you *have* to have sex." Well, they both got a really good laugh out of that, as did everyone else in the bank where she was parked at the drive-thru window. Her window was rolled down and the mic at the bank teller's window was on. An unintended stand-up routine was enjoyed by all.

Could it be that you are just too tired for sex?

Let's talk about sleep. Sleep deprivation can lead to serious health issues such as diabetes, cancer, cardiovascular disease, or obesity. As we discussed earlier, sleep deprivation can also affect anxiety and depression or even play a role in your lack of desire or sex drive.

There are multiple reasons that you may be suffering from insomnia. Other than stress and anxiety during the perimenopausal years, as hormones change, this can have an impact on your sleep. Estrogen and progesterone levels decrease. Progesterone is a hormone that promotes sleep. When your hormone levels are constantly shifting, this can cause disruptions in many areas of your life, including the ability to fall asleep.

Most women that I see in my health coaching business complain about either their insomnia, interruption of sleep, or general lack of sleep. Many have come to realize that their diets, and more specifically, what they are drinking is leading to insomnia and sleep disruptions. The main culprits are wine and caffeine. I can hear you now, "DON'T MAKE ME GIVE UP MY WINE!!" Women tend to think of wine as a stress reliever. Having a glass of red or white in the evening (or even two or three) makes them more relaxed. This could be true in the short term where drinking alcohol may help you fall asleep. But what often occurs is a disruption of your REM cycle. The more you drink, the more pronounced the effect is. So what exactly does this mean? Your REM sleep is restorative. Research shows that alcohol causes disruptions in sleep, especially in the second half of the night. This can lead to daytime drowsiness and poor concentration, along with lack of sleep.

Caffeine, of course, is a well-known stimulant. Drinking caffeinated beverages can lead to insomnia or sleep disruption, anxiety, nervousness, and in menopausal women, it can also trigger hot flashes. If you are suffering from any of these symptoms, it is best to stay clear of caffeine.

So just how can you be sure to get those ZZZ's and enjoy or desire sex?

- Maintaining a regular bed and wake time should be of the utmost importance.

- Create a relaxing bedtime routine such as taking a bath, personal skin care, listening to music, or having a hot towel scrub.

- Be sure your sleep environment is dark and quiet as well as comfortable and cool. This includes your mattress and pillows.

- Use your bedroom only for sleep and sex. Maybe keep the TV turned off (or remove it). Be sure those phones are NOT IN THE ROOM.

- Do not eat at least two to three hours before your regular bedtime.

- Exercise regularly but avoid it a few hours before bedtime.

- Avoid caffeine and alcohol close to bedtime as they can lead to sleep disruption later in the night.

Instead of a glass of wine in the evenings, I have discovered that herbal teas (no caffeine!) are extremely satisfying. They are flavorful and often soothing and relaxing. Some of my absolute favorites are spearmint, peppermint, ginger, hawthorn and hibiscus, or chamomile and lavender. A nice cup of herbal tea can help you to wind down before bedtime. Another soothing and immune boosting beverage you may enjoy just prior to beddie-bye time is called Golden Milk, otherwise known as turmeric tea. This is a delicious mixture of turmeric, coconut milk, cinnamon, raw honey, black pepper, and either ginger powder or a piece of fresh ginger. See the recipe below:

GOLDEN MILK

Serves: 4

Ingredients:
2 cups coconut milk (or almond)
1 teaspoon turmeric
Cinnamon, to taste
1 teaspoon raw honey or maple syrup
Pinch of black pepper (increases absorption)
Tiny piece of fresh peeled ginger root, or ¼ teaspoon ginger powder
Pinch of cayenne pepper (optional)

Directions:
Blend all ingredients in a high speed blender until smooth.

Pour into a small sauce pan and heat for 2-4 minutes over medium heat until hot but not boiling.

Drink immediately.

Another way to find some relaxation is to take a magnesium supplement. This is a great supplement to take for relaxation as well as stress relief. A fantastic way to add some magnesium into your life is to take a relaxing Epsom salt bath. Add a bit of organic lavender essential oil and your body will be cooing with appreciation. A warm bath just before bed time might just do the trick! Taking a daily magnesium supplement will also help to keep your body relaxed. Dr. Joseph Mercola, one of the top health experts in the country, refers to magnesium as "the missing link to better health." Dr. Mercola says, "Magnesium is perhaps one of the most overlooked minerals. This is especially important because an estimated eighty percent of Americans are deficient in it. The health consequences of deficiency can be quite significant, and can be aggravated by many, if not most, drug treatments." As with any supplement, always check with your healthcare provider before taking it. I would suggest, however, that every woman (and man) look into this beneficial mineral; I would go so far as to call it a miraculous mineral. You will be amazed at how many aspects of your health could be helped by taking magnesium supplements.

If you are having bouts of insomnia and you just can't turn off your mind, melatonin may help. Melatonin is a natural hormone that assists in regulating sleep habits. It is produced by the pineal gland at the base of the brain. You can also purchase it over-the-counter in supplement form. It is helpful for mild or occasional menopause induced insomnia and recent studies claim it to be a potent antioxidant and anti-aging therapy that has been shown to help prevent or treat multiple medical conditions including migraines. Check with your healthcare provider before using melatonin as it could interfere with blood sugar in diabetics as well as meds for high blood pressure. It could also make depression worse. Usual dosages range from .03-5.0mg to promote sleep with doses between 1-3mg being most common.

What is your routine two to three hours prior to bedtime? Are you literally wired? If you are on your computer, tablet, phone, reading device, or watching TV within a couple of hours of hitting the sack, you are possibly contributing to your sleepless nights. Those lights that are being emitted from these devices are tricking your brain into thinking it is still daylight, which in turn, blocks the melatonin from doing its job of making you tired and sleepy. It is best to make the two hours before bedtime a tech-free time zone and instead create a relaxing ritual, such as reading a book, taking a bath, or journaling.

Now that we may have conquered your sleep issues, what about SEX? Or were you hoping we'd just skip over that part? I think we sometimes forget what pleasure we derive from the close intimate contact with our dearly beloved. Our minds are somehow conditioned to think of it as a chore to be fulfilled rather than experiencing the enjoyment of fulfillment! There is joy in sex! We are sexual beings. Remember the romance? The courtship? The pleasures? How *happy* it made you? You *can* get your *happy* back! Your significant other will most definitely get *their* happy back too! Women will ask me, "How do I get my husband to leave me alone? How do I get him to require less sex??" I think the way to approach this is for *you* to require more sex! You deserve it! You deserve to desire it! While researching holistic ways to boost libido, one in particular caught my attention: "Make sex a priority." You heard that right. Evidently, during menopause, "without sexual activity, the vagina can become smaller and uncomfortably tighter." Say what?? Pain during sex is most definitely a big turn off and can lead to a lack of desire. Ultimately, this could affect your relationship. Throw in those bouts of night sweats and hot flashes and soon you are losing sleep and have become one fatigued chick! Your libido is connected to energy. If you haven't got any, you're probably not gettin' *any!*

Some great holistic ways to help with sex after menopause include the following:

- Communicate with your partner. Let them know if you are in pain. For vaginal atrophy and dryness, try using a natural lubricant like organic virgin coconut oil. It doesn't contain any preservatives or added ingredients. It is also anti-fungal so it can help keep yeast infections at bay. Why not spice things up ahead of time and use it as a massage oil too?! Just to be sure neither you nor your partner are allergic to it, test it on a less sensitive area, like your arm or leg. *Note: Don't use it with a condom, however, as coconut oil may break down the integrity of the condom. You can also try organic water based lubricants if coconut oil is not your thing.

- Try to remember that your largest sexual organ is your brain. Yup! Your desires, fantasies, and sexual stimuli can be triggered through scents and visuals, so be sure to spice things up with candles, essential oils, or anything you can think of that might trigger a *happy* outcome!

- Sexual intimacy can do wonders for your sex life. Just plain old hugging, hand holding, caressing, kissing, and sensual play are all wonderful ways to take it up a notch in your love life! I am a firm believer in hug therapy. There is proof that hugging boosts your helpful hormones! Not only that, but hugging also reduces the level of harmful hormonal effects! Research has shown that cortisol (the stress hormone) levels were significantly reduced in women during hugging sessions. The best news was that oxytocin (the pleasure hormone) was markedly increased between couples who hugged! Who doesn't enjoy a little more pleasure?! I just LOVE hugs!

• Reduce the stress in your life. One major contributor to low libido is a stressed out body! Reducing stress in our lives should be of the utmost importance to us as women.

• Eliminating or at least reducing your night sweats and hot flashes will most definitely help you get a good night's sleep, and thus allow you to have more energy for sex.

• Spend time on foreplay. Put less focus on intercourse and have fun with your lover. Give each other a massage for starters. This will give you that close intimate contact, along with being a fantastic stress reliever. Try a foot rub too! Maybe take a bath together. Add some candles and essential oils. These essential oils may help awaken the love bug: rose, neroli, fennel, ylang ylang, clary sage, jasmine, sandalwood, clove bud, or patchouli.

• Kegels! These are exercises to strengthen your pelvic floor muscles, the muscles that form a "sling" that hold your reproductive organs in place. When you have a weak pelvic floor, this can lead to incontinence or the inability to control your bowels. You can do Kegels anywhere! In the car, standing in line, or while getting your nails or hair done. Often times, your pelvic floor is weakened due to weight gain, pregnancy, childbirth, or simply aging. If the muscles are weak, then your organs could lower into the vagina. The exercise is a simple tighten and release method. The tricky part is finding the correct muscles to use. One of the best ways to do this is by inserting a clean finger inside the vagina and tightening your vaginal muscles around it. Another good way is by stopping your urine flow. However, don't use the urine method as a form of exercise, use it simply to find the right muscles. Always empty your bladder first before doing your Kegels. Practice makes perfect! So begin in private and find a quiet place to sit or lie down. Once you've got them down pat, you can do them anywhere! To begin, tense the muscles in your pelvic floor for a count of three, then relax them for a count of three. Repeat until you have done ten repetitions. Each day, increase the amount of time you hold your muscles tense until you can do it for a count of ten. Set a goal of doing three sets of ten repetitions every day.

Give it some time for the Kegels to work. It could take months before you notice a difference. Also, be cautious. You should not feel pain when doing your Kegels. If you are experiencing back or abdomen pain, then you are doing them incorrectly. When you are contracting your pelvic floor muscles, your back, abdomen and back muscles should stay loose. As with anything else, don't overdo it! We want those muscles to be strong, not tired!

So just how do Kegels help with your sex life? Well, these are the same muscles that are responsible for the contractions you feel during climax. They tone and strengthen your vaginal muscles, which can increase your arousal, as well as causing a tighter grip during lovemaking and more intense contractions during orgasm. YES! I'll have what she's having! Yowza! I see Kegels in your near future!

- Be sure there aren't any other medical conditions that may not be linked to menopause that could be causing your low energy and drive. Some possibilities could be low iron or an under active thyroid. If you happen to have been prescribed an antidepressant for hot flashes (many women are), some may cause your libido to diminish. Try a holistic method to try to combat the hot flashes before you switch to another medication. Always check with your doctor first before stopping or starting any medications or supplements.

- If you find that you are at a point where you are struggling in your relationship and need to address other concerns before making the sexual part work, I can't say enough about the benefits of couples counseling.

- The good news is that with a healthy lifestyle, including plenty of exercise, fresh air, staying hydrated, and eating a healthy whole food diet, you can make great strides in balancing your hormones and improving your love life.

Quite possibly, the lull in your love life is not directly associated with menopause or your menopausal symptoms. Could it just be that you've fallen into a boring routine at this stage of your relationship? Much like every aspect of our health, it takes some work to make it good. It takes a bit more work to make it great. Thankfully, it is doable! Look for different ways to spice it up. A romantic getaway or date might just be the ticket! How about a nice hot bath together? Maybe just some good old hug therapy is in order. Set a time to just cuddle and hug. Begin with hugging for two minutes without talking. Each day, add another thirty seconds to one minute. See where this leads you. Remember, no talking. Just hugging! I think you will be pleasantly surprised.

Especially when we are talking about your love life, spicing it up can be a lot of fun! It can, quite honestly, be *magical!* I want you to remember that you are worth every last second of experiencing the fulfillment and joy of a satisfying, pleasurable, and magical love life.

Now go and make the stardust happen!

CREATING MAGICAL MOMENTS

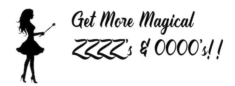

Get More Magical
ZZZZ's & OOOO's!!

So how is your sleep? _____

_____

_____

_____

What is your pre-bedtime routine? _____

_____

_____

_____

What could you change to help get better sleep? List three things you can start doing tonight!

1. _____

2. _____

3. _____

And your sex life?_____

_____

_____

_____

What could you do to make it better? List three things you can start doing today!

1. _____

2. _____

3. _____

GRATITUDE JOURNAL

_____

_____

_____

_____

_____

_____

_____

_____

_____

_____

_____

_____

_____

_____

_____

_____

_____

_____

_____

_____

_____

_____

_____

_____

_____

_____

_____

_____

_____

_____

_____

_____

_____

_____

_____

_____

_____

_____

_____

_____

_____

_____

_____

_____

_____

_____

_____

_____

SIX

Detox: Tech & Otherwise

Get rid of the crud! What is that you say? It is time to say goodbye to all of that tech stuff that takes up your precious time and wreaks havoc on your precious soul, as well as the stuff in your gut that may be contributing to some unhealthy symptoms causing your body to be out of balance. A great way to get rid of the crud is to do a detox where you can cleanse your body of these toxic and unhealthy substances.

As far as this chapter is concerned, we will apply both of these to what it is I wish for you to eliminate or substantially reduce in your life to help you get your *happy* back. So, you may ask, just what does this have to do with being a menopausal woman? Unfortunately, in this fast paced world that we live in, women often have way too much on their collective plates. As a menopausal woman, adding to the normal stress of career, family, household, finances, and fitting in time for a social life are the added burdens of unbalanced hormones, brain fog, and lack of exercise. Throw in a digital addiction and you've got a menopausal mess. Your hormone imbalance could already be providing you with anxiety, depression, and insomnia. These are also symptoms of technology addiction. There are physical symptoms as well such as weight gain or loss, carpel tunnel syndrome, head, neck and backaches. Why would you want to add to or compound the symptoms you are already trying to reduce?

According to the International Journal of Neuropsychiatric Medicine, one in eight Americans suffer from problematic internet use. About six to ten percent of iPhone users display signs of this addiction. Causes of addiction may be linked to a combination of biological, environmental, and genetic factors. Your technology addiction could, in fact, be working against your efforts to reduce your menopausal symptoms. Thankfully, there are ways to add peace and harmony to your life in a way that may seem hard at first, but ultimately, is so beneficial to your wellbeing.

First, let's start with the crud inside your body. Specifically, what I'd like to discuss is your gut. The crud in your gut. Perhaps you've heard the saying, "Listen to what your gut is telling you." Did you know that your gut is the control center for your physical and mental health, and that about seventy percent of your immune system lives in your gut? An unhealthy gut can lead to imbalances in your body, including hormonal ones. There are trillions of bacteria in your gut that are responsible for processing your food, providing a strong immune system to fight diseases, and for producing nutrients. Having a healthy gut is all about finding balance. What you eat, drink, and think effects what is going on in there! There are ten times more bacteria in your gut than there are cells in your body. You can apply the 80/20 rule here. About eighty percent of bacteria in there should be good and about twenty percent bad. In this scenario, your body is in a pretty healthy state. You will feel great with good energy levels and rarely get sick. Your good bacteria are working well, assisting with your digestion, crowding out the bad guys, producing certain hormones, vitamins and nutrients, as well as helping to keep your immune system working well.

So just what happens when you aren't eating a healthy, whole, and balanced diet? The bad or harmful bacteria can lead your gut on the path to illness and disease through inflammation, depression, infections, digestive issues such as constipation, autoimmune diseases, headaches, candida, hormone imbalances, and more. Your gut acts as your second brain. If your gut is unhealthy, it could affect your mental health, and vice versa. According to Kris Carr, health guru, "Your two nervous systems have an intricate relationship that's just now being explored by scientists through the field of neurogastroenterology. While the enteric nervous system initiates and sustains digestion on its own, signals from the brain, such as stress and anxiety, can have dramatic effects on how well it works. In addition, the brain receives chemical messages from the gut, which can affect your mood and emotions. In fact, the vast majority of serotonin (a neurotransmitter that regulates mood, sleep, anxiety, depression and more) is actually made in your gut, not your brain! It's all connected and sadly, few doctors ask you about your digestive health when you tell them you're feeling too blue to cope."

So just what can you do to maintain a healthy gut? Here are easy steps to keep the little guy happy and working at an optimum level:

- Eat a healthy, organic (as often as possible) whole food based diet.

- Take a probiotic supplement daily. This will help boost the good bacteria in your gut. I really like Dr. Ohhira's by Essential

Formula. You can find some good ones at your local health store or Whole Foods.

- Reduce the stress in your life.

- Eat both pre-biotic and pro-biotic foods:

Pre-biotic foods feed and support the growth of good bacteria. Some good ones to include are raw or cooked onion, raw garlic, raw leek, raw dandelion greens, raw Jerusalem artichoke, and bananas.

Pro-biotic foods are foods that contain large amounts of good bacteria. Some good ones are fermented vegetables like sauerkraut and pickles (in brine, not vinegar), kimchi, miso, kefir (made from cow's milk, it tastes like a liquid yogurt, but contains a far larger range of good bacteria then yogurt does), and coconut kefir. You may want to experiment with making some of your own!

You may also want to try making some healthy bone broths. These are quite healing to a distressed gut! See my Resource Guide for some recipe books.

- Remove or reduce processed foods, refined sugar, and environmental toxins from your life.

- Be sure to drink lots of filtered water! It is so important for your gut and overall health to stay hydrated!

What about the other crud in your life? The crud described as "nonsense." I like to think of this as the things we do in our lives that we know are not usually beneficial, often addicting, yet never easy to stop. Some examples of these behaviors are watching hours of the boob tube, including DVRing hours of our "favorite" shows to then sit and watch in marathon form, getting lost in Facebook posts (I am guilty!), spending hours with our chins almost embedded in our chests as we check our phones (often ignoring those around us, especially our loved ones), or playing silly games like Candy Crush, Angry Birds, or the new phenomenon, Pokémon Go! There are definitely positive elements of technology, from keeping us connected with others to the ease of information and knowledge at our fingertips. However, for many of us, none of this is done in moderation. All of this technology is wreaking havoc on our minds and bodies. You may be suffering enough with your menopausal symptoms. Let's not add fuel to the fire.

How do you know if you are tech addicted? Well, if you have anxiety when you leave your phone at home by accident, text while driving, constantly check Facebook, emails, texts, and are basically looking at a screen more often than not on a daily basis, then you probably have a tech addiction problem. If you notice that it is causing relationship issues, you probably have a tech addiction problem.

What about your sight? Too much screen time is responsible for blurry vision, eye strain, and dry eyes. Dry eyes are already a symptom of menopause. All of this can also increase those headaches. Then there are the mental effects of too much screen time. All that Googling can cause anxiety. There is actually a term for folks who are doing searches online for symptoms they may be having: cyberchondriacs. They are searching for ways to self-diagnose health problems. Quite possibly, this is you as you search for help with all of those annoying symptoms you are experiencing! This, in and of itself, can cause major anxiety. Other studies indicate that excessive social media use may increase stress levels. These are all things that women who are already experiencing menopausal anxiety, depression, and stress can do without in their lives.

Other ways that too much tech is messing with our mental flow includes sleep issues. Too much social media is linked to loneliness. Tech addiction can lead to withdrawal symptoms, and most disturbingly, studies show that too much technology is literally rewiring our brains, between the multitasking and the addiction we feel when we're without it.

If you really want to make a change in your life, and truly want to be of healthy mind and body, tech detox is a necessity. If you seriously want to get your *happy* back, breaking the transmitters that bind you begins today.

Let's begin your digital cleanse or detox. This may be very hard for you. I'd like to begin with a story one of my menopausal friends shared with me.

MENOPAUSE MOMENTS

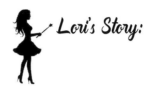 Lori's Story:

"Almost each morning, I log onto my computer to check my email. Usually, I have at least one or two notes in the back of my mind that I need to send to people about various things. So I log on, see that I've received a couple of emails, read them, respond if needed, and promptly log off. Of course, I've forgotten the reason I logged on in the first place and still need to send those one or two notes to people about various things. So, I log on, see that I've received a couple of emails, read them, respond if needed and promptly log off. I've again forgotten the reason I logged on in the first place and still need to send those notes to people. So I log back on, notice that I've received a couple of emails, read them, respond if needed, and log off. By golly if it doesn't occur to me that I've forgotten the reason I logged on in the first place and still need to send those same notes. So I log back on, see that I've received a couple of emails, read them, respond, and promptly log off…see my problem?"

———

I am sure many of you can relate to Lori. How much time do we waste perusing our email or getting caught up on Facebook, only to realize we've forgotten what we were supposed to be doing?

I mentioned earlier that one of the benefits of technology was being able to connect with people. While this is a fantastic way to stay abreast of those weddings, births, promotions, cat videos, and pics of delicious food, we must remember that it is more important to connect with the people in our immediate vicinity and to be present in each moment of our lives. In fact, it is crucial to make the person you are with the most important person in the world at that very moment. How often have you felt an irritation when you are enjoying someone's company and they receive a phone call or text which they immediately take, making you feel like the most ignored person in the universe at that exact moment? I'm sure we are all guilty of being that person who answers the call.

In a recent article in Psychology Today titled, *Are you Here? The Importance of Being Present* by Samantha Boardman, M.D., there is something called the *iPhone Effect*. Evidently, you may think you are being consciously polite and attentive by turning your phone over and turning off all notifications, however, if your phone is in sight, it can still be a distraction. "In an experiment with 200 participants, researchers found that simply placing a mobile communication device on the table or having participants hold it in their hand was a detriment to their conversations. Any time the phone was visible, the quality of conversation was rated as less fulfilling when compared to conversations that took place in the absence of mobile devices." The article went on to describe how especially detrimental this was to family relationships. "When children see their parents constantly on the phone, it sends a message about priorities." How often do you find yourself looking down and missing what is right in front of you? What message does it send to your loved ones when your eyes are drawn to your screen rather than their baseball game, dance recital, or gymnastic routine? How do you think they may feel when they look over at you to potentially see a proud smile on your face, but instead see you looking at your lap?

Here are seven steps to help you step away from the devices, reduce your menopausal symptoms of anxiety and depression, do a digital detox, and reconnect with those you love:

1. Put your phone AWAY. Don't plop it down on the table or anywhere in sight. Turn off all notifications. Agree to only check it in an EMERGENCY.

2. Take all devices out of your bedroom. Promise yourself to sleep device-free. As a matter of fact, put away all screens by 8pm each evening. Give your brain time to unwind before hitting the sack.

3. Choose humans over devices. Go to a coffee shop to connect with a *friend* rather than the free *Wi-Fi*. Disconnect to reconnect.

4. Limit your social media time. Did you know that the more time a person spends on Facebook, the less satisfied they are with their own life? Find apps that can help you track and limit your time (ironic, right?). There are apps which will block you from using social media if you're not "scheduled" to.

5. Is there an old hobby, activity, or passion that you've long forgotten about? One that brought you joy? Pick it up again by putting down the device. How about a good book? Or maybe you've always wanted to try a new hand at painting, singing, or playing an instrument? Replace the handheld device with a racket, paint brush, or guitar.

6. Try and go a whole day without looking at any devices. The weekend may be a good place to start.

7. And finally, experience the joy of being present in each moment of this magical life you have. Maybe even leave your phone home on a Friday evening date. Gaze into each other's loving eyes instead of a cold blue screen.

There is a quote I love in an article titled, *What is Being Present?* "Being present is what we experience when we are completely at peace with this very moment. It is a life journey where we constantly grow our inner peace."

Wishing each of you a magically happy, peaceful, ever present, and crud-free life!

CREATING MAGICAL MOMENTS

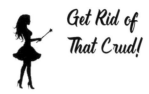

List three ways you can eliminate the crud in your gut beginning now!

1. _____

2. _____

3. _____

List three things you can do to reduce/eliminate nonsense tech/ device time today:

1. _____

2. _____

3. _____

GRATITUDE JOURNAL

_____

_____

_____

_____

_____

_____

_____

_____

_____

_____

_____

_____

_____

_____

_____

_____

_____

_____

_____

_____

_____

_____

_____

_____

_____

_____

_____

SEVEN

Queen of Sandwich

The sandwich generation. Being in the middle. There are over seventy-four million baby boomers living in the U.S. today. That is approximately one-fourth of the U.S. total population (per the 2012 census). These are the folks born between 1946 and 1964, more than half of which are women. According to nabbw.com (National Association of Baby Boomer Women), by the year 2030, over fifty-four percent of boomers will be women. That makes for a whole lot of changing hormones in the universe at one time. The term "sandwich generation" is defined as a portion of the population who may still be raising children under the age of eighteen or supporting their grown children while also caring for their aging parents. While the financial responsibility itself can add a level of stress to an already stressed out life, imagine what the emotional, and ultimately, physical effects are on a person of the sandwich generation.

A recent article in Psychology Today, *Being in the Sandwich Generation,* presented some interesting facts: "While balancing the double burden of caring for parents and children at the same time is hardly new, improvements in geriatric care are ensuring that people are living longer. That means that adult children often carry this burden decades longer than their parents or grandparents did. The stress that this places on adult children acting as caregivers can be overwhelming, especially as new health problems develop in their aging parents." Add to this the fact that close to thirty percent of young adults aged 25-34 still live with their parents due to lack of employment, and you can imagine how the stress levels can skyrocket. According to CaregiverAction.org, sixty-six percent of these caregivers are women with an average of twenty hours per week being spent on caregiving.

You wonder why women suffer from anxiety, depression, and adrenal fatigue? The majority of these women are between the ages of 40-59, prime menopause years. Perhaps this describes you? While dealing with your own uncomfortable symptoms of hot flashes, mood swings, and fatigue, you may also be tending to an aging parent who needs constant care. How much can one body take? You probably feel as if you don't have the time to care for yourself, or you may have forgotten the importance of doing so. Self-care is a matter of survival.

Caregiver stress is real and can lead to our own health issues if we don't find ways to cope with it. What can you do as a menopausal Queen of Sandwich to alleviate caregiver stress?

1. Let's begin with taking care of your own health. If we can keep ourselves in optimum good health, it will afford us the ability to be a strong support system to our loved ones, both older and younger. Follow the strategies throughout this book to keep in top form. Self-care can take the form of eating healthy, exercising, going on a social outing, getting plenty of sleep, as well as

using stress reducing techniques like getting a massage, meditation, or yoga. This also includes taking breaks from your care giving role. Maybe even schedule a respite stay for your parent for one to four weeks to give you time to recharge. Remember, you are not being selfish. Self-care is an absolute necessity. Try to do at least one special thing for yourself each day.

2. Plan Ahead. Know what your parents' wishes are, financially as well as medically. A great resource to help your parents organize is *The Drop Dead Book* by Preferred Living Solutions (see my Resource Guide). This comprehensive resource includes sections for insurance policies, medical history, financial information, usernames and passwords, social security cards, warranty information, and much, much more.

3. Attend seminars that deal with the issues your elderly parents may be facing, like dementia or Alzheimer's.

4. Find support groups in your area. Venting can be quite helpful.

5. There are multiple local agencies you can contact for help. A great source for finding the help you need is AgingLifeCare. org. Here you can find info on working with an Aging Life Care professional, otherwise known as a geriatric care manager. They are experts in guiding families as they care for their loved one through assessment and monitoring, planning and problem-solving, education, advocacy, and family caregiver coaching. This allows for the families to ensure quality care for their loved ones. These professionals are health and human services specialists who act as guides and advocates for families who are caring for older relatives or disabled adults. Be sure to

utilize the expertise of a care manager or specialist.

6. If your children are living with you, be sure that they pitch in at home. As teenagers growing up with my grandmother living in the cottage in our backyard, my sisters and I were often tasked (along with our daily chores of laundry and cleaning) with taking my grandma grocery shopping and to her doctor's appointments. It was just part of life. We had two parents who worked full time. We all pitched in where we could. Remember the old saying, "It builds character!" If you have siblings that live close by, be sure they are helping you share the load as well. Be specific and tell those who offer to help exactly what it is they can do. Keep a running list to delegate. This might even include running an errand for YOU, so that you are better able to be present for your loved one.

7. Prioritize. Make a list of all that you need to accomplish. Let go of those items that are not of immediate necessity.

8. Be present. You may be struggling to keep it together and things may seem overwhelming. Beyond overwhelming. Having to care for an elderly parent is stressful. There is no doubt about it. I am asking you to find the joy in each moment. If we focus on the good moments, the time we are sharing with them, maybe retelling some stories or just giving them a long bear hug, showing them how much they are truly cared for, the love and care you have for your parents should not only comfort them, but it will bring you an abundance of grace and peace. Everyone can get a little bit of their *happy* back!

CREATING MAGICAL MOMENTS

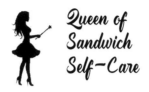

What can you do to alleviate caregiver stress?_____

_____

_____

_____

_____

_____

List at least one thing for each day of the coming week that you can do FOR YOURSELF. Remember to put YOURSELF on the calendar each week from now on.

Monday:_____

Tuesday:_____

Wednesday:_____

Thursday:_____

Friday:_____

Saturday:_____

Sunday:_____

Queen of Sandwich

GRATITUDE JOURNAL

_____

_____

_____

_____

_____

_____

_____

_____

_____

_____

_____

_____

_____

_____

_____

_____

_____

_____

_____

_____

_____

EIGHT

Get Your Happy Back!!

You picked up this book because you felt a need. The need may have stemmed from the numerous menopausal symptoms that were driving you crazy! The hot flashes, mood swings, or annoyingly dry vagina!! It may have been because you are in the midst of menopause and you are feeling down, maybe a little anxious and depressed. You may be unhappy with your weight and energy levels. You want that magical fix! You so desperately want to GET YOUR *HAPPY* BACK!! Darn it! You want to LIVE the LIFE you CRAVE!!! You've made a commitment to yourself that you will do whatever it takes to live life to its fullest, healthiest, and as stress free as possible!

You most definitely do not have to live with the uncomfortable symptoms of a "typical" menopause. There are multitudes of holistic remedies within these pages and at your fingertips. You may never need to reach for a pharmaceutical again. I've provided you with some basic holistic yet effective ways to achieve good health, a calm mind and body, balanced hormones, a purpose to your life, and good (if not great) sleep and sex! It's time for you to take action.

My wish for you is that through the guidance of *The Magic of Menopause,* you can accept that you are strong, beautiful, and filled with passion and purpose. Rather than let the social stigma of being a menopausal woman define your experience, I want you to embrace every last bit of it. These can be your "freedom" years. You are free of having a period, free to have all the sex you want with no chance of pregnancy, free to pursue new goals and dreams, free to take care of you! With one third of your life ahead of you, there is plenty of time to do anything you put your mind, body, and soul to!

This is your life and only you can live it. Through taking the steps to get your life and hormones in balance, you will discover your own true magic. Remind yourself about what is good about yourself. Treat yourself lovingly and with kindness.

Remember the acronym we talked about? H.O.P.E. Have Only Positive Expectations! Come on! Put on those Pollyanna rose-colored glasses! It is good for your health!! Your menopause years can be the happiest of your entire life.

I am your menopausal fairy godmother. I have given you the tools (stardust) you desire and need to live the most wonderfully magical life you could imagine. Imagine your life free of hot flashes, irritability, anxiety, and those extra pounds. Imagine a life filled with more energy, more sex, and more happiness! It is truly up to you now. I could inundate you with inspirational quotes like, "Where there is a will there is a way," or, "The secret of getting things done is to act," but as I have lived and learned and guided and observed, there is one quote which I know holds true for each and every one of you magnificent women:

"You've always had the power my dear,

you just had to learn it for yourself."

-Glinda, The Good Witch

I think Glinda would agree that there can be magic in menopause….

Cheers & Love,

Lorraine

Your Menopause Fairy Godmother

CREATING MAGICAL MOMENTS

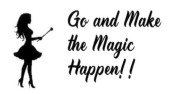

Go and Make the Magic Happen!!

Insert your name is a fabulous woman who deserves to live a magical life! The time is NOW to make it happen! I am becoming the woman I've always wanted and was meant to be!! I will live a magical life!!

Repeat loudly and often!!

GRATITUDE JOURNAL

_____

_____

_____

_____

_____

_____

_____

_____

_____

_____

_____

_____

_____

_____

_____

_____

_____

_____

_____

_____

_____

_____

_____

Resource Guide

BOOKS:

Allergy Exclusion Diet:

The Allergy Exclusion Diet by Jill Carter & Alison Edwards

Gut Health:

The Body Ecology Diet by Donna Gates & Linda Schatz

Beauty/Self-Care/Supplements:

The Truth About Beauty by Kat James

The Magnesium Miracle by Carolyn Dean

The Wisdom of Menopause by Dr. Christiane Northrup

Inspirational:

One Thousand Gifts by Ann Voskamp

The Power of Intention by Dr. Wayne Dyer

Eat That Frog by Brian Tracy

Hay House

Bone Broth Recipes:

Nourishing Broth: An Old-Fashioned Remedy for the Modern World by Sally Fallon Morell

Bone Broth Secret: A Culinary Adventure in Health, Beauty, and Longevity by Louise Hay and Heather Dane

APPS:

Meditation/Health/Self-Care:

Stop, Breathe, Think by Tools for Peace

Plant Nanny (reminder to drink water)

SKIN CARE:

SunshineBotanicals.com

Neal's Yard Organics: https://us.nyrorganics.com

SUPPLEMENTS:

Magnesium: CALM by Natural Vitality or Doctor's Best High Absorption 100% Chelated Magnesium

Probiotic: Dr. Ohhira's Probiotics by Essential Formula

Phytoestrogen: A-Ma-Ta TM by Dr. Christiane Northrup: http://a-ma-ta.com/index.php/dr-northrup

ANTIOXIDANTS:

Pycnogenol: http://www.pycnogenol.com

Ubiquinol (CoQ10) with Resveratrol: Reserveage Ubiquinol CoQ10 with Resveratrol (You can find it at Whole Foods or Amazon.com)

WEBSITES:

Anxiety/Stress: Calm Clinic: http://www.calmclinic.com/

Elimination Diet: WebMD: http://www.webmd.com/allergies/guide/allergies-elimination-diet

Essential Oils: Mountain Rose Herbs: https://www.mountainroseherbs.com/

Meditation: The Art of Living: ArtofLiving.org

Skincare Database: Environmental Working Group: EWG.org (Skin Deep)

Volunteering: NationalService.gov

CAREGIVER INFO:

The Drop Dead Book by Preferred Living Solutions: http://preferredlivingsolutions.com/the-drop-dead-book/

Geriatric Care Manager: AgingLifeCare.org

Works Cited

Aboujaoude, E., Koran, LM., Gamel, N., Large, MD., Serpe, RT. "Potential Markers for Problematic Internet Use: A Telephone Survey of 2,513 Adults." *National Center for Biotechnology Information (PubMed - indexed for MEDLINE),* 11 Oct 2006, Web.

Allsworth, Jennifer., Cooper, Amber., Grindler, Natalia. "Persistent Organic Pollutants and Early menopause in U.S. Women." *PLOS One,* 28 Jan 2015, Web.

American Cancer Society. "Breast Cancer." *American Cancer Society, Inc., 1*8 Aug 2016, Web.

Beyond Celiac. "Non-Celiac Gluten Sensitivity." *Beyond Celiac,* n.d., Web.

Boardman, Samantha. "Are You Here? The Importance of Being Present." *Psychology Today,* 1 Oct 2015, Web.

Bryant, Alison. "7 Amazing Benefits of Joining a Club." *allwomenstalk,* n.d., Web.

Caregiver Action Network. "Caregiver Statistics." *CAN,* n.d., Web.

Carr, Kris. "How to Improve Your Gut Health." *Crazy Sexy Wellness, LLC,* n.d., Web.

Cirino, Erica. "Can you Drink During Menopause?" *Healthline,* n.d., Web.

Demiralp, Emre., Jonides, John., Kross, Ethan. "Facebook Use Predicts Decline in Subjective Well-Being in Young Adults." *PLOS One,* 14 Aug 2013, Web.

Gorman, Rachael Moeller. "New Science Links Food and Happiness." *Eating Well,* May/June 2010, Web.

Grens, Kerry. "When Removing the Uterus, Leave the Ovaries: Study." *Reuters,* 22 Mar 2013, Web.

Howard, Jacqueline. "This is How the Internet is Rewiring Your Brain." *The Huffington Post,* 22 Feb 2016, Web.

IARC. "Press Release N° 240: IARC Monographs Evaluate Consumption of Red Meat and Processed Meat." *World Health Organization.* 26 Oct 2015, Web.

INH. "Processed Meats Too Dangerous for Human Consumption." *The Institute for Natural Healing,* 21 Jul 2015, Web.

Kohn, David. "When Gut Bacteria Changes Brain Function." *The Atlantic,* 24 Jun 2015, Web.

Kraft, Sheryl. "Menopause and Anxiety: What's the Connection?" *Healthy Women,* 9 Aug 2011, Web.

Laughlin-Tommaso, Shannon. "Diseases and Conditions: Menopause." *Mayo Clinic,* n.d., Web.

Mann, Denise. "Alcohol and a Good Night's Sleep Don't Mix." *WebMD,* 22 Jan 2013, Web.

Mayo Clinic. "Drugs and Supplements: DHEA." Mayo Foundation for Medical Education and Research, 1 July 2014, Web.

Mercola, Joseph. "Magnesium—The Missing Link to Better Health." *Dr. Joseph Mercola,* 8 Dec 2013. Web.

Mercola, Joseph. "Are Probiotics the New Prozac?" *Dr. Joseph Mercola,* 25 Jul 2013, Web.

Myers, Amy. "Thyroid Health Part III: The Toxin, Heavy Metal, and Thyroid Connection." *Amy Myers MD*, 31 Jul 2015, Web.

Nature's Health Foods. "Ubiquinol." *The Pro-Fit Group,* n.d., Web.

Northrup, Christiane. *The Wisdom of Menopause: Creating Physical and Emotional Health During the Change.* Bantam, 2012. Print.

Porter, Valencia. "5 Natural Ways to Balance Your Hormones." *The Chopra Center,* n.d., Web.

Pote, Kaitlyn. "Menopause Around the World." *Women in Balance Institute,* n.d., Web.

Present Living. "What is Being Present?" *Present Living & Learning, Inc.,* n.d., Web.

Rodriguez, Diana. "Maintaining Your Sex Drive During Menopause." *Everyday Health,* 1 Dec 2014. Web.

Vitelli, Romeo. "Being in the Sandwich Generation." *Psychology Today,* 26 Jan 2015, Web.

Writing Group for the Women's Health Initiative Investigators. "Risks and Benefits of Estrogen Plus Progestin in Healthy Postmenopausal Women." *The JAMA Network, JAMA.* 2002;288(3):321-333, Web.

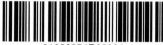

91666554R00091

Made in the USA
San Bernardino, CA
23 October 2018